TABLE OF CONTENTS

INTRODUCTION
IN THE BEGINNING: P3 – P9
THE START OF THINGS TO COME: P10 – P19
WHEN DOUBT ARISES: P20 – P34
HOW TO RE-FOCUS YOUR LIFE: P35 – P44
ALMOST THE END: P45 – P59
SURVIVING THE FIRST RADIATION: P60 – P73
THE SECOND ONSLAUGHT: P74 – P89
MORE MEDICAL BLUNDERS: P90 – P102
FIGHT YOUR OWN CORNER: P103 – P116
THE SEARCH CONTINUES: P117 –P130
RUNNING OUT OF TIME: P131 – P145
THE CUTTING BEGINS: P146 - 157
FINALLY HOPE FROM DARKNESS: P158 – P172
ANOTHER RAY OF HOPE: P173 – P183
I WAS CORRECT AGAIN: P184 – P192
NEVER GIVE UP: P193 – P202
THE SUN SHINES ONCE MORE: P203 – P209

This book is dedicated to my family who have also been on this long journey with me and to those who became dear friends that I met along the way, some who have sadly lost their own life's journeys to this awful disease. I have chosen to write this book after being asked on numerous occasions by friends to share my own personal cancer journey to others, after being delivered a very frightening Stage Four terminal cancer diagnosis and an expectation of no more than three months to live in September 2014. I have decided to fulfil these requests and to tell my story of a personal cancer struggle after receiving a terminal diagnosis in 2010, brought about from shocking medical negligence. I hope that from reading my own personal story that it may just offer help, support, and inspiration to others, who may be walking along a similar pathway as mine, and may the sun always shine ahead of you on your road.

Strength doesn't just come from winning
Your struggles develop your strength
It's when you go through hardships and you decide
NOT to Surrender, then that's real strength

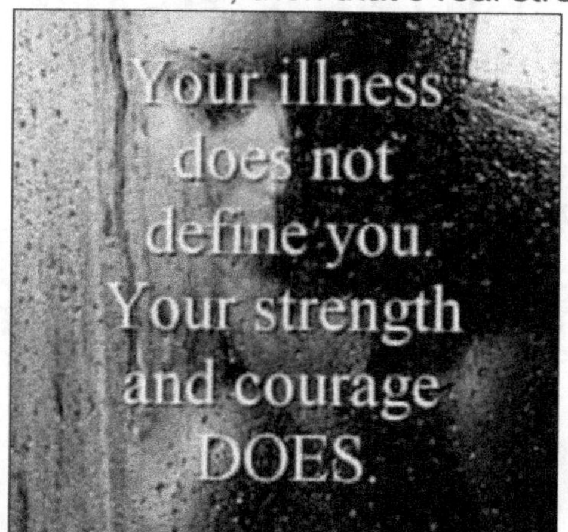

The cover picture location is Moneycarragh Road near Castlewellan, County Down in Northern Ireland, where my father used to walk his horses.

IN THE BEGINNING

If you are ever in any doubt about anything that you have heard, or you aren't quite sure about something that you have been told, then you should always consider seeking a second opinion. If you are still not sure after receiving a second opinion, then you should look at getting a third one.

In 2008, I was employed with a well-known Australian bank, as one of their team of investment specialists. I had an investment target to reach each month of over one million dollars and a client base totalling over four hundred investors. I always managed to achieve my monthly budget, but even with my consulting work of more than forty hours each week, it was almost virtually impossible to properly look after, maintain and service these four hundred clients. I was the bank's number one investment specialist in Australia. I had previously received several awards from various financial institutions, for providing financial planning advice and in 2005 I received a national award for producing the best Financial Plan in Australia. This was presented to me at a gala dinner held at the Old Customs House in Brisbane city, and which was sponsored by BHP, a very large Australian mining company.

On any given day, whilst working for the bank, I barely managed to have a proper lunch break. Even on a Friday afternoon after all the other investment specialists finished work for the week at lunch time to head off for refreshments, I would still be conducting customer interviews in my office until after 5.00pm. This was over an hour and a half after the bank had officially closed its business doors for the working day.

After four years of daily intense pressure, I made the decision to approach the senior management of the bank regarding my position, and I tried explaining to them what I considered would be a much better approach going forward for everyone concerned. I told them that most employees just decide to resign from their existing positions and leave the company (at this time I was continually being head hunted by other major banks) but I'm fair and honest and I would like to discuss a plan with you that might just help me to overcome my daily exhaustion, and were I would still be able to manage and maintain my existing client base of four hundred customers. I offered to continue to work for them from a small office at their regional banking centre located on the Sunshine Coast in Queensland, use my own motor vehicle and carry out regular home visits, as many of my clients were elderly customers and some found it very difficult to travel to their nearest bank.

The management suggested that I should give them six months in order to consider my plan. I told them that the current system they had in place was an unfair system, and the expectation of trying to achieve an investment target of over one million dollars each month, on top of trying to service an existing client base of over four hundred customers, was just simply not attainable.

I agreed to their six-month timeframe and their response was "Oh, in the meantime you can also train a new investment planner for us? They can sit in on your everyday client interviews as part of their learning curve." I replied "Now you are attempting to place even more pressure upon me at an already difficult time. I shouldn't have to train your employees for you.

4

You should be employing professionally skilled people to fulfil your banking roles, that are already qualified as investment specialists for each of their respective positions and roles. I should not be expected to also carry out a Human Resources role as well."

Unfortunately, after the six months timeframe had passed, nothing had changed at the bank, as I had basically become like an athlete, who had to keep winning their races for them. If, at any given time I dropped back to a number two position on their monthly 'League Ladder' which was made up from the bank's various investment specialists and their monthly achievement figures, I could expect to receive a phone call from my regional manager, asking me to explain what was going on and that I needed to get myself back up to the number one position on the bank's 'League Ladder' again as soon as possible. I later discovered that my performance figures impacted upon her bonuses as the bank's regional manager.

After the agreed six months period, I finally decided that regrettably I'd had enough, and I resigned my position as an investment specialist with the bank. I then made the decision that I would open my own small investment office nearby. I looked around Caloundra, where I worked on the Sunshine Coast in Queensland, to see what might be available to me, as I knew I would require good ground floor access, as many of my existing clients were quite elderly and some also had disabilities. I finally found some suitable premises that I was confident would be convenient for my clients. I agreed a monthly rent figure for the property with the landlords and very shortly afterwards I started to fit out the new office layout. I built a reception area, two client interview rooms, installed ducted air-conditioning and finally a small kitchenette at the rear of the building, as I knew my clients enjoyed a cup of tea or coffee served in a Royal Doulton cup and saucer during their appointments.

With the usual banking protocol in place at the time, I wasn't allowed to make any contact whatsoever, with any of my existing banking clients for a period of three months. This didn't really concern me at the time as they all managed to find me at my new office themselves, as the word got out around the town.

After a few months working in my new business role, I considered that now might be an appropriate time for me to start looking at setting up some personal insurance, in the event of any sickness that might occur to me in the future, especially even more so now, since I had become a one-man band financial specialist.

Shortly after submitting my personal insurance application, I received a request from the insurance company asking me to have some blood tests carried out, which I agreed too. I then arranged to have these blood tests carried out through my own GP. A few days after the test reports had been completed, my GP contacted me to advise that my blood results weren't that good, as he had found some things which concerned him and he suggested that it might be best if I didn't submit them to the insurance company straight away, but rather I should consider having some new blood tests carried out in a few weeks, to see if things had improved in any way. I followed my GP's advice and a few weeks later I had some new blood tests carried out, which unfortunately still showed up similar results to the previous ones. He then suggested that I should consider having a Gallium scan carried out, to try and identify what was going on inside my body at this time. The scan was subsequently arranged and completed at a medical facility on the Sunshine Coast, close to where I was living at this time.

After the report had been finalised, the results showed that nothing untoward was really going on inside my body at this time. The Gallium scan takes the form of a particular dye, which is injected into the body through a cannula needle, which is then inserted into either the left or the right arm. It is carried out inside a radioactive protected room of a building.

It just so happened that the medical facility that I was attending on this day, to have this scanning procedure carried out, was located on the ground floor level of a building, positioned below where my previous bank employer's regional office was located, at Kawana on the Sunshine Coast.

After several weeks things appeared to have returned to normal once again and my GP was confident enough, that my recent blood reports were now suitable enough to be submitted to the insurance company, who had originally requested them. The previous blood reports could have simply been showing up as some sort of infection, which had since disappeared. I submitted the requested blood reports to the insurance company and the cover which I had initially requested was established, soon afterwards.

Around six months later, one evening I was suddenly admitted to my local hospital at Caloundra, with what later turned out to have been a case of acute pancreatitis. After spending the night in the hospital's Emergency Department, I was then discharged several hours later, to return home again. The hospital's emergency doctor, who just so happened to have been one of my clients, told me that I should consider making an appointment with a local Gastroenterologist, who could check out, what was going on with me, as things didn't appear to be quite normal.

I accepted this advice, and I arranged a private appointment myself, and within a few days I visited a local gastroenterologist in Caloundra, where I was still living at this time. This specialist then arranged for me to have some CT scans carried out and then later told me "I think you have Lymphoma." I said "That's a cancer, isn't it? Are you sure? Could it not just simply be a case of Sarcoidosis instead?"

He replied 'No, I have seen similar images like this many times before on lots of CT scans." I was totally devastated to be told that I now had cancer, especially since the Gallium scan, I had conducted only two months earlier, had shown that there was nothing whatsoever was going on in my body.

How on earth could this happen to me so quickly? I left his clinic and returned to my new office suite where I had my receptionist cancel all my appointments for the remainder of the day. I shut my office door, sat down on my desk chair and I begin to sob. The Gastroenterologist then decided that he would refer me to another hospital nearby at Nambour, again on the Sunshine Coast and there the specialist that I saw decided that they would carry out a simple watch and observe approach. I thought this was a strange way to deal with a newly diagnosed cancer patient. I decided to discuss this with own GP, who also considered it to be a very strange approach indeed. Finally, after a few months, in a further attempt to confirm that this diagnosis was indeed correct and that I did have cancer, a procedure was arranged at the hospital, which would involve the removal of a lymph node from my stomach region for a microscopic biopsy. This lymph node would then be sent to the hospital pathology laboratory for further testing, to see if I did have cancer.

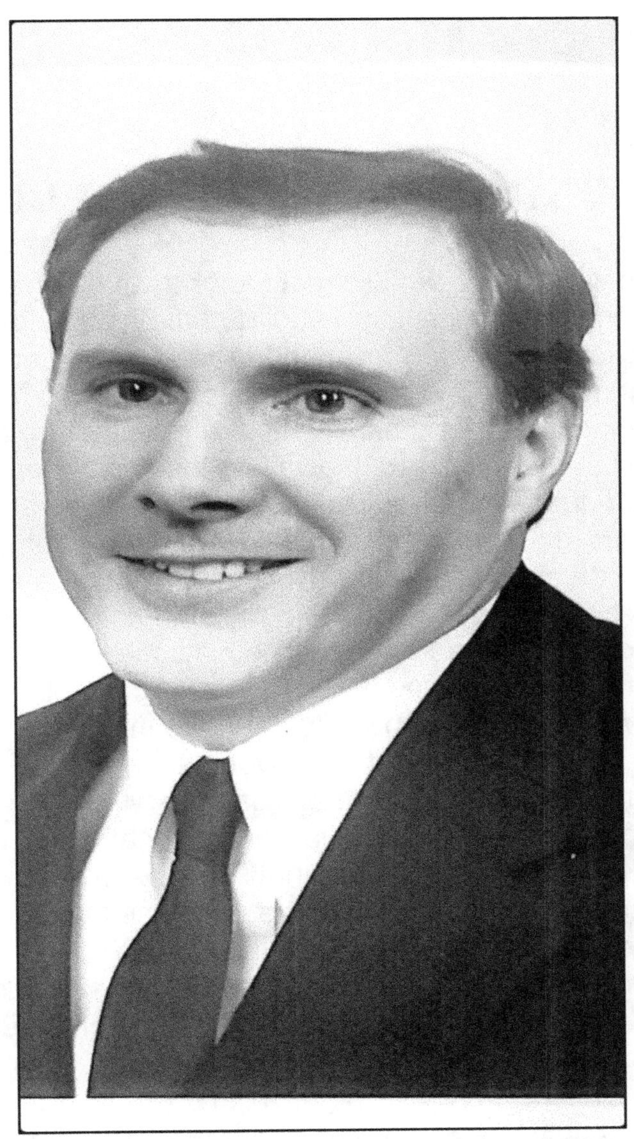

Robin 2005 in his Investment Specialist role

THE START OF THINGS TO COME

Well, this was what I would simply refer to as being a 'botch up' from the very beginning. I attended the hospital as planned, to have the pre-arranged procedure carried out of the lymph node removal. As was customary, I was then changed into the usual hospital attire for the theatre and placed on to the patient bed, awaiting the anaesthetist to arrive and deliver his sleeping potion to me. Once he had finished his infusion, I was then wheeled directly into the operating theatre nearby, to commence my procedure to have the lymph node cut out from my stomach. Suddenly I started to watch the surgeon cutting his scalpel through the centre of my stomach lining before inserting the black gas tubing, which he was then going to use to inflate my stomach up with, like a tent. This would then allow him to operate much more freely. I could see the whole procedure happening in front of me, as I lay on the theatre bed. The surgeon could very clearly see that I was watching him carry out the scalpel cuts and he told the anaesthetist who was still present in the theatre room at this time "You haven't given him enough, increase his dose" which he then did. After the anaesthetic was increased, I no longer saw or felt anything further with this operation.

Around one week later at home I started to develop what is commonly referred to as a "staph" infection. This is an infection that patients can sometimes pick up in hospital after a procedure has been carried out. I had somehow managed to contract this infection during my stay in the hospital and my stomach had now swollen up like a pregnant lady. I was now in a lot of pain and discomfort.

A few weeks later, after I had started to show signs of recovering from the "staph" infection, I returned once again to the hospital at Nambour, to be delivered the results of the lymph node pathology biopsy testing.

The surgeon who had carried out the previous procedure brought me into his office and then proceeded to tell me "Well, we did the biopsy as you already know, but unfortunately we removed a piece of your normal tissue and not the actual lymph node, that we really wanted to remove for the biopsy, but on the bright side of things we did however manage to fix up your hernia on the way out of your stomach." I couldn't believe what I had just been told. What a botched procedure from the very beginning. The surgeon then said what I had already heard before "We will just keep an eye on you for the time being." I then asked him if there had been any signs showing, of anything going on inside my stomach, to which he replied, "Oh yes, we believe that you do have Non-Hodgkin's Lymphoma, but we will just watch it for now." I left the hospital very clearly in a state of shock and total disbelief after being told this.

I then made the decision that I needed to remove all this stress, which I had been clearly suffering now for many years, and to get myself out of my current employment position. The world's global financial crisis (GFC) had just started and stock markets around the globe were plummeting everywhere. Anyone holding any investments whatsoever were all being affected, and many banks were almost ready to collapse. The world was in a total panic mode, and it was a very nervous time for anyone holding any type of investments and even those holding cash deposits in all the major banks, seemed to also be at a great risk. It was certainly a very difficult environment for any investment specialists to be operating in.

I decided that I would contact the Financial Licensee, under whose investment licence I was currently operating at this time, to explain my recent health issue.

They were most helpful and later assisted me to find another investment specialist, who would be able to take over my existing business and who could look after my clients. I was devastated and very sad to have to do this, as I had developed great rapport with many of my clients, many of whom had also become close friends, that I helped outside of normal business hours, even with teaching some of my more elderly clients how to use a computer. I had even enrolled many of them into tuition classes at their local libraries. I had managed to establish a regular income to live from, and to help support my family with.

Despite all this, I felt that it was the right thing to do for my own health and general well-being and that I should now begin to focus on my life from a different approach, without the constant daily stress and pressure, which I had been enduring now for quite a considerable number of years.

After several months of attending the usual appointments at the hospital with one of the Haematologists, a role which I later discovered, is only a blood specialist and not a cancer oncologist. I asked my own GP if he could refer me to a proper cancer oncologist. I was then referred to an oncologist within the same hospital, however, sadly I underwent the same lack of response each month as I had previously experienced with the original Haematologist.

The usual blood tests that never seemed to change very much, except to show elevated liver enzymes. On one occasion when I attended my usual hospital appointment my medical records file couldn't be found anywhere in the clinic.

The receptionist searched within the cancer department. I asked the oncologist about my recent blood results, only to be told "I'm sure they will be fine."

The oncologist I was attending and who had also become very familiar with my previous experience in finance, then said to me "How about we just talk about finance instead, shall we? I've been watching the shares of this company on the ASX (Australian Stock Exchange) what do you think about them?" At this same moment the office door was knocked and one of the reception ladies entered the room carrying what later turned out to be my missing hospital records file.

The oncologist asked the lady "Where did you find this?" To which she replied, "You left it in the toilet's doctor." The oncologist then thanked her, and she left the room. At this point I said, "So that's what you think of my present medical condition, you just simply dump my medical file in the hospital toilet and then decide to discuss finance with me instead."

I was now starting to become very disillusioned once again, at the lack of response I was receiving from this hospital oncologist. I arranged another appointment with my own GP to discuss with him my ongoing concerns. At this appointment I suggested that maybe I should be referred to a different hospital in Brisbane city for another opinion. A lady who I knew at this time had previously been treated in Brisbane for her breast cancer, so my GP assisted me with a referral to her cancer specialist.

Unfortunately, this specialist's field of expertise was confined to dealing with breast cancers only and he referred me instead to another specialist, who was a colleague of his, and who dealt primarily with Lymphoma and Leukaemia diseases only.

13

It was only much later that I discovered once again that this specialist was also only just another Haematologist and not an Oncologist, specialising in dealing with specific types of cancers.

I met this doctor in late 2009 and I discussed with him about the botched surgery, that I had previously experienced at the hospital in Nambour, and that up to this point I have been told I have a Non-Hodgkin's Lymphoma cancer, but it has never actually been proven or confirmed to me, so as far as I'm concerned that's based on an assumption only. I'd like it to be proven to me by a proper procedure and pathological laboratory testing for my own peace of mind. He accepted my request and agreed to arrange another procedure for me, only this time at the hospital in Brisbane, where I had now started to attend. My liver enzyme readings at this time were still very high so it was decided that I should have a liver biopsy procedure carried out first, before arranging any lymph node removals. This is where part of the liver is sliced away and then the portion that has been removed is sent for pathological testing in a laboratory, using various staining methods.

Well, the liver being the largest organ in the human body, it most certainly does not like to be chopped up in any way. The pain was horrendous, and I was constantly on morphine every hour for almost twenty-four hours. It was so painful that I could hardly breathe most of the time.

It later turned out to have been caused by internal bleeding from the liver being dissected. I can normally handle quite a lot of pain, but this was a very tough one indeed. It felt so bad that as I continually tried to breathe, I thought that several of my ribs had been broken during the procedure and the treating team then agreed to send me to the Medical Imaging Department, to have further X-rays carried out of this region.

I was taken to this department of the hospital on my bed, for the X-rays to be carried out, to see if they could find out what the problem might be, that was causing me to endure such horrific pain.

After this X-ray procedure, pathological testing and staining was completed, the liver biopsy result came back from the laboratory as being normal. Nothing could be found, and it was then put down to being some sort, of an inflammation or infection, possibly being caused by a virus. I personally suspect that it could have been related to the previous "staph" infection that I had contracted at the hospital in Nambour several months earlier.

Still searching for answers, it was agreed to carry out another operation at the hospital to remove a Lymph node, once again from my stomach region for further pathological testing. I was really hoping that this next planned surgical procedure would be more successful than the previous operation had been.

I was trying very hard to feel confident that the lymph node which had been selected from the scans for removal, would indeed be the lymph node they would be able to remove, for the pathology testing to be completed a second time around.

This time the anaesthetist managed to inject me with the correct dosage of anaesthetic, which then put me to sleep very quickly, allowing the operation to take place, without me watching it again live, which I had managed to do before when the last procedure was carried out at the hospital in Nambour. It was later confirmed that the Lymph node had indeed been removed this time, as planned.

It was now March 2010 and almost nine months had passed from when I had originally been told that I had cancer, but in fact nothing had been confirmed up to this point. I now had to wait several more weeks on the pathology results coming back from the laboratory.

The wait once again became a very concerning and distressing time. I travelled back to the hospital in Brisbane once more, and as I walked down the long corridor to the cancer department, I stopped for a few moments to admire the beautiful paintings which adorned both sides of the corridor walls.

It had become a regular habit of mine on each hospital visit and before any of my scheduled appointments with the specialist, to do this.

I found it very calming and therapeutic walking down this long corridor, which I had now done previously, on so many occasions towards the cancer department. It always reminded me of a Johnny Cash song, that he sang many years ago called "I Walk the Line."

It was beginning to feel a bit like this now each time I made this long walk down this corridor towards the hospital lifts, which then took me upstairs to the cancer department on level four. This very sadly, was to become a regular trail of mine, I got to know very well over the future years, from my regular monthly attendances there.

The only part that I enjoyed about walking down this long corridor leading to the cancer department, was stopping to admire these walls, as they were always beautifully adorned with personal paintings of all various types, that skilled artists had finished in oils, water colours and pencils.

Each trip I made there, the pictures had always been changed over from my last appointment and new ones had reappeared as replacements.

I always found this very relaxing at a very stressful time. Even if only just to stand in the corridor for a few minutes and admire the skills of so many other very talented people. I found it very calming and relaxing before reaching the cancer department. Sadly, this was always a very depressing and sorrowful place, to have to attend and to see people who you knew, weren't going to be able to make it, and who would very soon become victims of this horrible disease.

Things were to start to change very dramatically after this. At this meeting with the specialist I was informed, that yes, we do believe that you have a very low-grade form of a Non-Hodgkin's Lymphoma cancer.

He then went on to tell me that there are two different types of Lymphatic cancers. There is Hodgkin's Lymphoma cancer which is very curable, and which can be removed through having a surgical procedure carried out, radiation and/or chemotherapy, and the other one is a Non- Hodgkin's Lymphoma cancer which is incurable.

"Unfortunately, we think that your type of cancer is the Non-Hodgkin's Lymphoma type. There is no cure for this type of cancer, but because we belief that yours is just a very-low grade form of Non-Hodgkin's Lymphoma, we will simply adopt an observe and monitor approach with you at this stage."

"This is normally a cancer that most people usually die with, and not a cancer that many people actually die from."

I asked the specialist if he could be any more specific regarding this type of cancer and if it would be possible to receive some further information, to try to help me understand it a little bit better please?

He then drew me a set of steps on a piece of scrap paper he had sitting in front of him on his desk. He told me "You are here on the very first step of these stairs. You have a very low-grade type of cancer which we will simply monitor on a regular basis every few months, but if it gets any worse in the future, then at this stage of the stairs (which he then drew again on the same piece of scrap paper) we will offer you some form of chemotherapy. However, after this there is always a possibility that within five to six years after you receive the chemotherapy treatment, that you might be required to have Stem Cell treatment, in order to be able to continue to survive."

Again, this was devastating news, but I had finally received confirmation of what was going on inside my body, as I had now been waiting anxiously for almost twelve months, to receive this news. Even though it was very depressing to be told this, I now felt a little bit more relieved, knowing that I had been able to receive an outcome, albeit not the best outcome that I wanted to receive, but it was now a result. The very sound of the word chemotherapy I had always associated with horror stories and bad reports, and it frightened me immensely when I heard it being discussed at any time. The word itself stood for 'chemical therapy' and that to me seemed to indicate toxicity to the human body. For the next six months I regularly attended the hospital to have follow up blood tests completed, that remained unchanged from month to month and the specialist advised me on each of my visits, that he would be pleased just to continue with an observe and monitor approach with me for now.

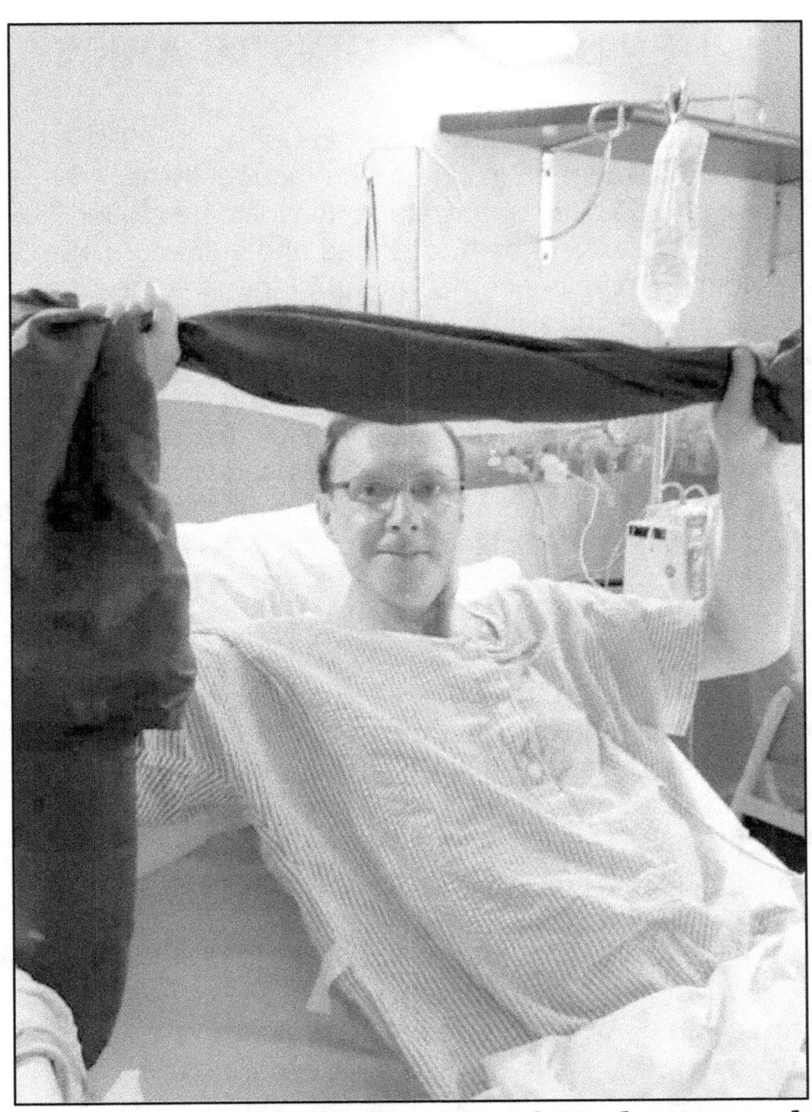

Robin preparing for the Lymph Node removal

WHEN DOUBT BEGINS TO ARISE

At my next scheduled appointment in September 2010, I once again asked the specialist if he thought I was continuing to go okay at this stage, to which he replied "Yes, everything appears to be unchanged and quite normal, you have nothing to be concerned about." I then left the appointment feeling a little bit more relieved, if only for another few months. At around this same time I needed to have an ear grommet fitted into my right ear as I had always suffered from what was known as a 'Glue' ear since my childhood. As a young boy my mother used to take me regularly on the bus, from our little village in County Down to Belfast city where I attended the Ear Nose and Throat Department of the Royal Victoria Hospital on the Falls Road.

I had also suffered Adenoid issues growing up as well. The reason the grommet had been fitted into my ear in the beginning was to help with the air flow through my ear as the Eustachian tube was partially blocked, resulting in a reduced air flow through my ear, which then in turn resulted in partial hearing loss issues. Each time the grommet had been inserted back into my ear again, it instantly relieved the hearing loss problem, and I was always able to hear much better once more. The issue with fitting ear grommets is that they always manage to work their way back out of the ear again at some point and need to be regularly replaced.

This was very important, especially as a child, when your mother gave you the all too regular warning to "do as you are told or else, you'll get the wooden spoon." I never really favoured this spoon offer, as a popular toy in those days.

20

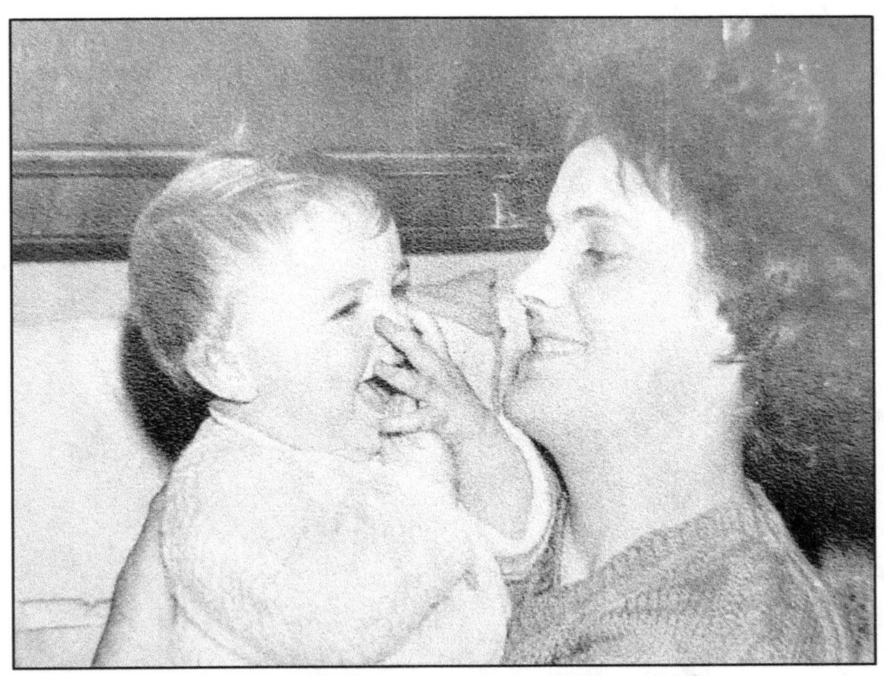

Robin with his mum at 12 months

Since first migrating to Australia in 1992 I had been attending an ENT (Ear, Nose and Throat) specialist on the Sunshine Coast in Queensland for many years, after my doctor had referred me to his clinic to have my ear grommet fitted, as I needed them replaced from time to time. My doctor even today in 2022, remains the very same doctor that I first attended when I arrived in Australia and for whom I have total respect for.

During one of these grommet procedures at the Buderim Private hospital in 2010, the ENT specialist, who was unfamiliar with my previous childhood medical history thought that my Eustachian tube blockage appeared to be slightly more prominent than it had been before.

He said that it was also very possible that he might not have noticed it on his previous examinations. He then forwarded his ENT report to the specialist that I was attending in Brisbane. The report stated, 'could likely be an Amyloid deposit.' I then started to research 'Amyloid' only to discover that it is a build-up of protein, normally associated with cancer. Upon hearing this latest development, I immediately decided that I would start investigating this further myself.

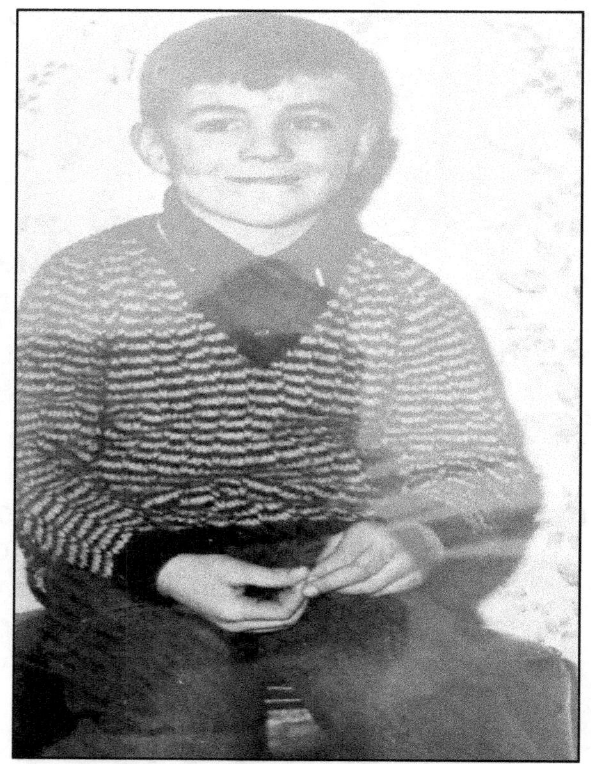

Robin aged 6 in Clough, County Down

I researched various medical centres to see which ones might be the best to have further explorations made. I paid privately once again, to have my own tests carried.

I wanted to see if there were any other traces of this suspicious 'Amyloid' tissue, anywhere else in my body. I had an 'Echocardiogram' completed. This is a specific test to check your heart and I also had further whole-body tests carried out.

After these tests were all completed, each individual report showed up that there was no Amyloid whatsoever in any of these tests. I told the specialist that I had attended the Royal Victoria Hospital in Belfast ever since my childhood. I was treated there for 'Glue' ear issues and my adenoids were also supposed to have been removed, when I was only nine years old, but the operation was later cancelled as it was deemed an unnecessary procedure at that time. I even remembered the name of the numbing spray that they inserted into my nose in the hospital back then and which, apparently is still in use today.

It was called Xylocaine. He said "Yes, that's correct, and we still use that exact same spray to this very day, both here in the clinic and also in the main hospital.'

The results of all these tests now provided further proof that there were absolutely, no other traces of this suspicious 'Amyloid' protein deposit, to be found anywhere else in my body, at this time.

In December 2010 I travelled back once again to the hospital in Brisbane to attend one of my regular scheduled appointments with the specialist. In the few months between having my last appointment, the specialist had now received a copy of the Ear, Nose and Throat Pathology report.

23

This was the report that had been prepared after the ear grommet insertion procedure had been performed at the Buderim hospital on the Sunshine Coast.

This type of ear grommet insertion takes the form of a 'T' piece and requires to be carried out in a hospital theatre under a full anaesthetic procedure.

The idea behind inserting a 'T' tube grommet into the eardrum, is that it is designed to be able to remain positioned within the eardrum longer, than just inserting a normal straight tube type grommet, that can usually work its way out of the ear much quicker.

After reviewing the recent report on his computer, the specialist then turned around from his desktop and shocked me by saying "Right, we might need to look at starting you on some chemotherapy." I was totally shocked at hearing this news. I immediately replied to him by questioning it, "But why would you need to start putting me onto chemotherapy at this time, especially considering that at my last appointment here at the hospital when I asked you if you thought I was going ok you told me that, "Yes, everything appears to be fine?"

He said, "I think that there might be a link now between your Non-Hodgkin's Lymphoma and this new recent discovery of 'Amyloid' deposit in your right ear."

I replied by telling him that "I'm not particularly happy at all about this. I have had all the tests completed privately that I felt were necessary to prove that there is absolutely no sign of any 'Amyloid' tissue showing up anywhere else in my body. I believe that the tissue, which is showing, to be blocking around my eustachian tube, that has only been noticed recently, has been there from my childhood days.

It's nothing new and the Ear, Nose and Throat specialist has also advised me, that it's quite possible that he might have missed spotting it on his previous examinations."

I told him that this was only an 'assumption' from the Ear, Nose and Throat specialist, as nothing had been removed for a biopsy, to test if it really was an 'Amyloid' deposit.

He then said that the only real way to find this out for definite would be to carry out what he called a Bone Marrow Aspirate. This is where a huge needle is inserted into your lower spinal region and sample cells are then extracted from the body's own marrow for pathological testing in a laboratory.

I agreed to have this procedure carried out at the hospital in order to prove to him, that having to start me on this new chemotherapy plan was totally unnecessary.

The following week I had the Bone Marrow Aspirate carried out, and which turned out to be an extremely painful procedure at the hospital in Brisbane, as had been pre-arranged by the same specialist. This procedure was very similar to having a hole drilled into your lower back with a battery-operated drill bit. My back remained very painful for quite a few days after having this aspirate carried out.

About a week after this procedure had been carried out, I received a call from the same specialist requesting to see me for a new appointment. I travelled back to Brisbane once again and at this appointment I was told, "Yes, we need to start you on chemotherapy straight away." Again, I was totally shell shocked to hear this latest news. I had always heard such bad reports about chemotherapy treatments, and I questioned it once again, as to why this was necessary for me at this time?

The specialist told me, that he would allow me to have my Christmas period with my family, but after this we needed to commence the chemotherapy treatment straight away in the New Year 2011. I didn't know what to say at this stage, but I asked him what type of chemotherapy was he planning to give me.? He said, that in this case it would be the less severe of the two chemotherapy treatments known as R-CVP and not the harsher version known as CHOP.

This is where my very first warning to readers begins.

At the time I did not request to review a copy of this report, as I honestly believed that what I was being told by the specialist must be the truth and that I had no other reason to doubt, it in any way. Very regrettably for me, it wasn't until nine years later in 2019, after I requested a copy of my own hospital medical records, that I managed to obtain a copy of the original December 2010 Bone Marrow Aspirate Pathology report. The report that I read at that time was extremely alarming and even today as I write this book, I still find it very difficult to accept, or to even try to understand, how this could happen to someone, that someone unfortunately at that time being me. I totally trusted and believed that what I was being told at that time was the truth, as to why I was being coerced into having chemotherapy that I knew I didn't want to have.

The pathology result from the Bone Marrow Aspirate from 10th of December 2010 that I discovered, read: -

'NORMAL MARROW'
'There is NO MORPHOLOGICAL EVIDENCE OF LYMPHOMA'
'There is NO MORPHOLOGICAL EVIDENCE OF AMYLOIDOSIS, in these specimens.'

haematopoiesis is present in normal proportion with normal morphology. There one large blood vessel present and a number of smaller ones. Congo Red and Crystal Violet stains show no evidence of amyloid deposition. CD138 positive plasma cells account for less than 3% of total cellularity.
RETICULIN: CityplaceNormal

DIAGNOSIS
Normal marrow - no morphological evidence of lymphoma. Correlation with flow cytometry is required.
No evidence of amyloid in these specimens.

The Bone Marrow result in 2010 showing no cancer, yet I was given 6 months of chemotherapy.

So, in fact what this Pathology report clearly showed, was that it was very evident at the time when the Bone Marrow Aspirate was carried out at the hospital in December 2010, that there was absolutely no evidence of any traces of cancer anywhere in my entire body. Why on earth would any 'specialist' prescribe chemotherapy to any patient, who, especially in my case very clearly didn't need to be given it? I recently read a report where a Doctor in Michigan in the USA was sentenced to forty-five years imprisonment, for prescribing unnecessary chemotherapy to patients, many of whom died after receiving it, and for no other reason than so he could receive huge commission payments from the various pharmaceutical suppliers, that he was dealing with at the time for selling their products.

It was a huge class action instigated by the families, as none of the victims even had any cancers to begin with in the first place. It had all been fabricated purely for financial reasons only.

After I continued to read my hospital medical history, it became even worse again. I discovered that the specialist had already checked my scans in December 2010 and as well as doing the Bone Marrow Aspiration, had also re-stained my liver, including doing urine tests and an echocardiogram, which I had already performed privately to check around my heart for any signs of Amyloidosis, and nothing had shown up anywhere. So, as well as having the Bone Marrow Aspirate results, he also had further proof in December 2010 that there wasn't any evidence anywhere of 'Amyloid' in my body. He was only basing the forced chemotherapy, that he was about to commence me on, based on an assumption from an Ear, Nose and Throat specialist.

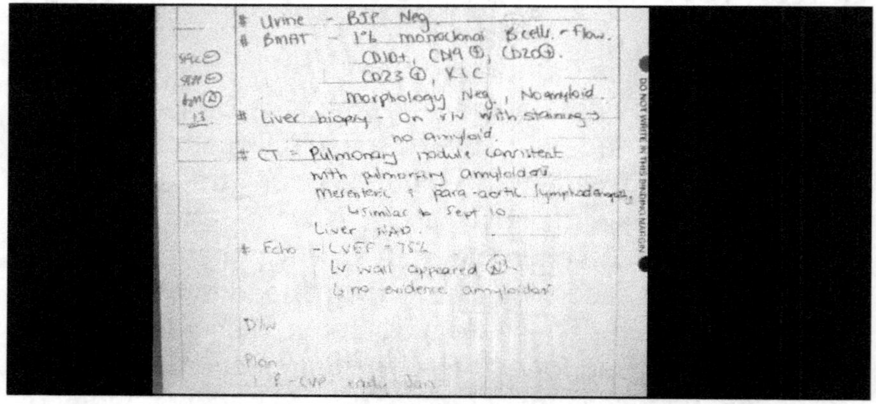

Further evidence from December 2014 of no Amyloid Cancer anywhere

Very reluctantly in January 2011, I made my way back to the hospital in Brisbane to commence the dreaded chemotherapy procedure, that I was told I must have.

This being the 'treatment' that I had originally feared the most along this dreadful journey so far and even then, I really felt like I was being coerced into having something that I shouldn't really be having and that I didn't need.

Even walking the line again down the hospital corridor to the Cancer Department, the walls of which were brightly decorated as always, with fabulous artworks I had a real sense of discomfort or 'gut feeling' at that time.

I didn't even know then, how much of our immune system is 'housed' inside our own gut. In reflecting then, even my body's own immune system was trying to warn me off from going through with this toxic poisoning.

Each chemical infusion day in the following five months of unnecessary chemotherapy poisoning, beginning in January 2011 was displaying all the signs to me, that the world was trying its very best to tell me that something was wrong in what was being inflicted upon me.

The very first infusion day beginning in January 2011 took over eight hours to complete, as my body kept continually rejecting the chemotherapy infusion and this 'chemical treatment' had to be stopped several times, due to extreme sweating and very severe heart palpitations my body was experiencing.

During this extremely long infusion period I was approached by a cancer care support officer who suggested to me that I should consider joining a patient chemotherapy support group.

She said that by doing so it might help me to share with others the ongoing side effects of the treatment, the emotional outcomes and any other related issues from the chemotherapy 'treatment'. I thanked the young support officer very much for this and I told her that it was something I would certainly look at considering later.

After only the first day I decided that this was not something I wanted to be a part off. For eight hours I had just listened to other patients sitting on each side of my hospital bed during my infusion, sharing their own personal horror stories regarding the side effects of this terrible treatment.

From how awful people were feeling, how some were considering suicide, to others asking me "How long did they give you to live? I've been told I have only about six months left, and even then, that's if I'm lucky."

The very first day witnessed the worst Brisbane flooding in many decades. I could not even get out of the city afterwards. I had to move from the hospital ward to a nearby motel room for accommodation, before I was able to travel back home to the Sunshine Coast a few days later, once the flooding started to subside and the main roads had been re-opened.

The next month in February, as I attended the second poisoning session in Brisbane, I watched the most horrific earthquake unfolding in the centre of Christchurch in New Zealand live on my television, which was positioned above my bed in the hospital ward. Then again in March, I had the third chemical infusion.

On this day another massive earthquake and tsunami had just taken place, totally devastating the entire coastline of Japan.

In April 2011, I received the fourth round of chemical infusions. This day witnessed the worst ever flooding in Tasmania in over a century. This was then followed by massive tornadoes in the United States of America. The universe was certainly trying to tell me that something wasn't quite right.

30

The last and final month of chemical infusions was one month later in May 2011 when this poisoning finally came to an end with the Royal Wedding of Prince William.

This was a sign that it was finally all over and a day that I was very glad to have managed to reach, as I had made it this far on the journey.

The saddest part of leaving the cancer ward on that day was when I asked one of the nurses what the ward next door housed, as I had witnessed several patients inside various incubation chambers. She told me, "They are the patients that are having stem cell replacement treatments and a place that you really don't want to be." I suddenly remembered the conversation that my specialist had with me several months earlier, when he told me that I too might probably require Stem Cell treatment within five to six years of being given chemotherapy. Sadly, I could clearly see that some of these patients were extremely ill, and I feared that this could also be a future outcome for me as well.

When it was finally all over, I was told by the specialist that I would be given a few weeks to allow my body to recuperate after all the chemotherapy that I had just been administered with. After this, it was then back once again to the hospital in Brisbane for yet another Bone Marrow Aspiration to be taken and then to await the results of the test from the hospital pathology laboratory.

At the end of June, I had yet another appointment scheduled with the specialist, to discuss the results of the most recent Bone Marrow Aspirate, the same specialist who had initially started this whole poisoning programme in the first place. It most certainly felt like the Johnny Cash song 'I Walk the Line' as I travelled down that same long corridor once again.

This interview with the specialist even today in my mind still totally shocks me, as I can still very clearly remember it being told to me.

I was told at that meeting "Sorry about that, but even though you didn't really need that chemotherapy in the first instance, I just decided that I would give it to you as a precaution, just in case you might have needed it."

From the pathology report that I have now received back from the laboratory, and which I have reviewed of your last Bone Marrow Aspirate, it would appear, that there has not been any change whatsoever in your 'Amyloidosis,' during this period, nor have we witnessed any further type of progression."

To be told that the treatment I had just received was totally unnecessary and not even required, left me in sheer disbelief and shock. How could this happen to me? To find out nine years later, that the results of the original December 2010 Bone Marrow Aspiration had shown that there was absolutely no evidence of any cancer in my body whatsoever, neither Lymphoma nor Amyloidosis, was a very harrowing and deeply disturbing discovery.

One thing that I did discover by accident whilst enduring this toxicity, was that even though most people who receive this toxic 'treatment' automatically lose their sense of taste and discover that they only have a metallic taste in their mouth, I discovered that I was able to taste blueberries.

I have shared this information with many other people since then and they have also told me that they too have had similar experiences with being able to taste blueberries.

I was then told that I should continue to have regular blood tests performed every few months and to keep going with my regular reviews with the specialist.

At no time, was I ever told that my original Bone Marrow Aspirate in December 2010 and the hospital Amyloid scans, had shown that there were absolutely no signs of any cancer activity in my entire body. For several years I continued attending the hospital in the belief that I still had cancer throughout my body and that within the next few years, I too would probably require to have Stem Cell treatment, for me to be able to continue to survive, which was what I had previously been told in 2010.

I decided in advance, that the most appropriate preparation I could now make, expecting that this might occur within the next five to six years, as the specialist had warned me, might be the case, would be to relocate from the Sunshine Coast, where I had lived for the past 20 years and to reside closer to the hospital in Brisbane city for convenience.

Sadly in 2012, I moved from the Sunshine Coast to Burpengary, which was then only a thirty-minute drive to Brisbane city, compared to over an hour's drive from the Sunshine Coast. For the next few years, I came to terms with the fact that I was trying to deal with an incurable cancer and that I would try to stay as positive as I possibly could.

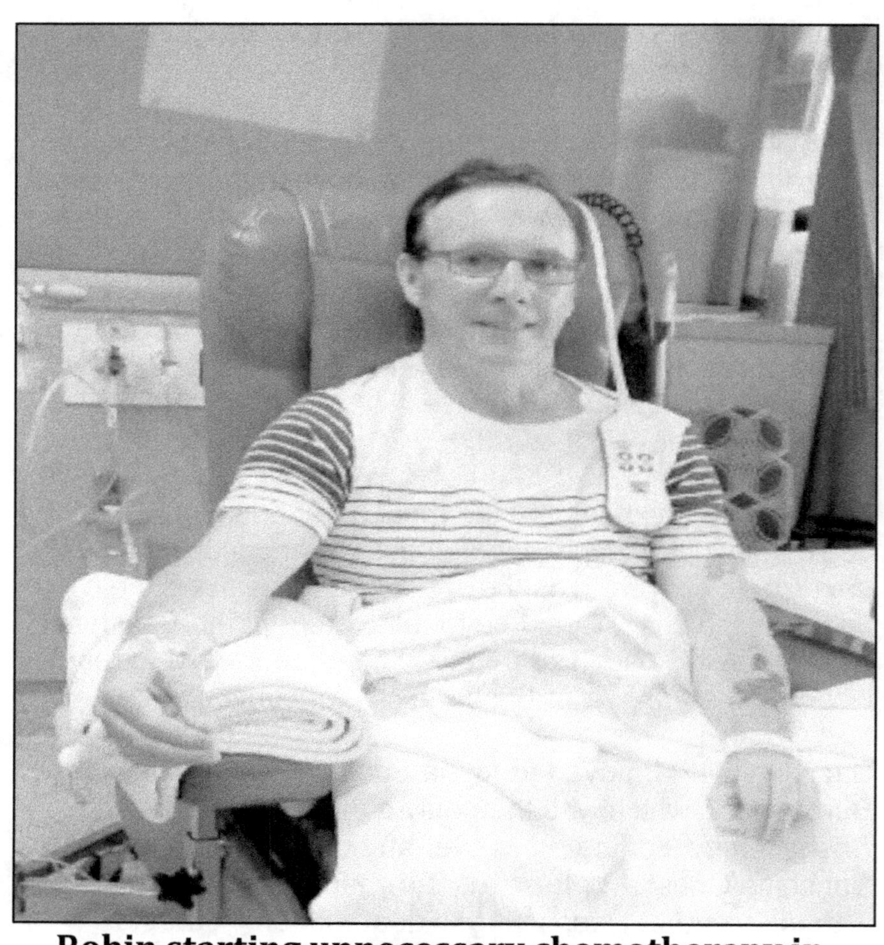

Robin starting unnecessary chemotherapy in January 2011

HOW TO RE-FOCUS YOUR LIFE

I made up my mind that now was the time for me to start to focus on the things in life that I enjoyed doing the most. I decided that I would commence doing some car restoration work and especially Ford Escorts, which had been my very first car as a teenager. I looked up welding classes on the internet and I enrolled at the Technical College in Nambour for weekend training in learning how to MIG weld. The teacher in the classroom had only one arm and he was a brilliant welder. It was further proof to me that in life we all have choices that we can make. We can either Give Up, we can Give In or we can Give it ALL we've got. I finished this course at the college within a few weeks and I purchased my first small welding machine and I continued to practice my welding skills at home, until I felt confident enough to proceed with restoring my first car.

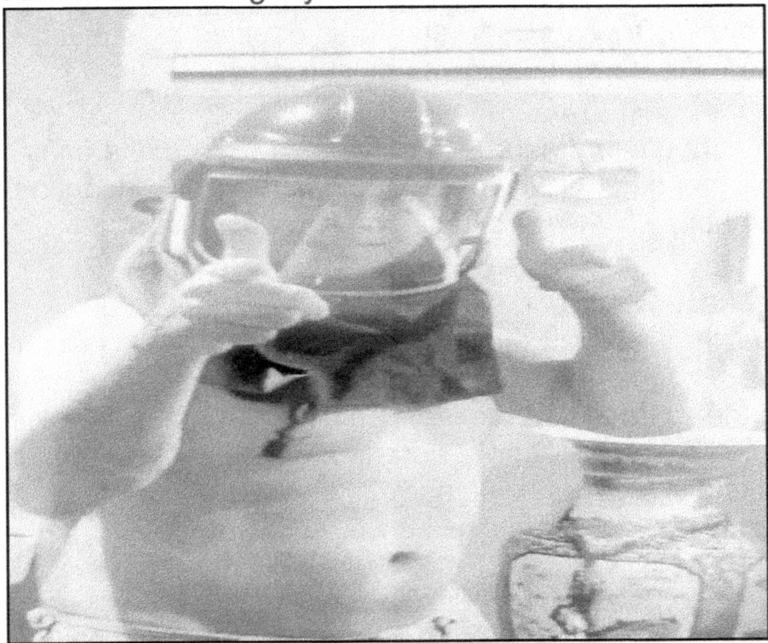

Robin with his Welding helmet

I also started to study auto-electrics and I learned how to manufacture the various wiring looms and components that were necessary to completely wire a vehicle from the very beginning until completion. Over the next ten years I designed, restored, raced and sold ten of these cars. All of which later appeared in articles of various newspapers and magazines throughout both Australia and in the UK. It was from these cars that I developed, that I became well respected around the country for my workmanship, and which I believe I have still retained to this present day. During this same period, I also continued each day to study health and well-being.

I was still quite concerned now about what damage the chemotherapy might have had upon my body.

I certainly wasn't aware at this time about the Bone Marrow Aspirate results, as this was only something I was to discover nine years later after I had decided to request copies of my own hospital medical records.

I spent hours and hours each day researching, starting early in the morning until it was time to commence working in my workshop, which was situated next to my home.

I purchased and read, volumes of medical books and health magazines, as well as continuing to carry out my own online research. One magazine which I had managed to obtain was the world-renowned New England Journal of Medicine for medical professionals. I started to read some of the older versions of the magazine as well as some of the most recently published editions as well.

One edition was from 2009. This was only just one year before I was first told that I needed chemotherapy by the specialist, from the hospital in Brisbane.

Whilst reading this edition I discovered an article relating to Non-Hodgkin's Lymphoma patients who had been given R-CVP chemotherapy and how they could develop secondary cancers later in life after this treatment was finished. The first of which was normally skin cancer, and the deadliest form of all, being the skin cancer Melanoma. This totally horrified me as to why would any patients be given chemotherapy, if it would indeed cause them to get cancer from it several years later.

This didn't seem at all possible and neither did it really make any sense to me, but to see it now being printed in the most highly acclaimed medical journal in the world, must surely mean that there must be some substance to it, otherwise it would not have been featured as an article, in this very prestigious magazine to begin with.

I decided that I would continue with my own personal research as I was now beginning to become more and more disturbed with what I was discovering each day.

In June 2014 I attended another appointment with the specialist at the hospital in Brisbane. I voiced my concerns to him at this time about some of the recent discoveries I had made during my research activity. I mentioned to him about the secondary cancers that were caused by the chemotherapy drugs R-CVP which he had given to me. I was politely told that this claim was pure rubbish. I said "Why would the most highly acclaimed medical journal in the world make up that claim if it could not be substantiated? It just did not make any sense."

I told the specialist that I would like to have a whole-body scan completed at this time, to review the current state of my entire body and to provide me with some peace of mind, as what I was reading was beginning to alarm me.

My request was immediately refused, and I was then told
that this would be a complete waste of money and that it
was totally unnecessary and not needed. I said
nevertheless, I would prefer to have one please as it might
just provide me with some comfort if I did have it. Again, my
request was refused, and I was told again that it was a
totally unnecessary procedure.

The next part that I am about to tell you about, was in my
own opinion something of a miracle that saved my life in the
first instance. Early one morning in August 2014 I had just
commenced my daily routine in the workshop. My wife drove
into the driveway nearby. It was around 8.00am and I
wondered where she had gone to, as I had not heard her
leave the house earlier. I asked her where she had been to,
so early in the morning? She had a friend who travelled
around Australia as a clairvoyant, and she had recently
renewed contact with her.

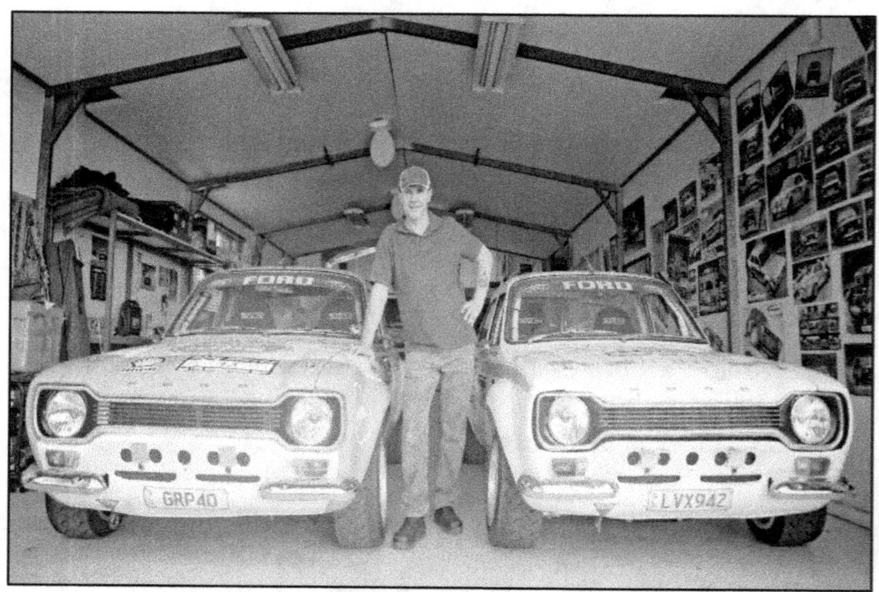

Robin in the workshop with the Ford Escorts

She told me that as she was passing through that morning, she had managed to catch up with her in a local park for a coffee and a chat. I said that was very nice and how was she going.? She replied that she was fine.

She then asked me when was I due to have another appointment again with the specialist in Brisbane?

I said that I already had another one scheduled in a few weeks' time and why do you ask me that? She replied that her friend Ashana had told her that there was something going on inside my stomach, to which she replied that we already knew that from the Non-Hodgkin's Lymphoma biopsy report they said was in my stomach. She said, "No it's got nothing to do with that, there is something else going on and I think that he should get it checked out as soon as possible."

I said "I can't just go the hospital and tell them that I want a body scan based on what a clairvoyant has just told you, but I will ask again anyway, as I had already requested a scan when I had attended my last appointment, however it had been refused and I was told that it was a totally unnecessary procedure and a complete waste of money.

In late August 2014 I had the next scheduled appointment at the hospital in Brisbane. As I walked along the corridor once more, decorated with all the freshly displayed paintings that I always took the time to admire, I thought to myself that it seemed highly suspicious as to why I was being denied a check-up scan. Was it because something might just be discovered? At this appointment I told the specialist that if he couldn't arrange for me to have a whole-body scan carried out at the hospital then I would arrange to have one carried out elsewhere and I would pay for it myself.

He said, "You don't want them as they will give you too much radiation." I said, "I don't care at this point, as I would really like to put my mind at ease with what is actually going on inside my own body."

Finally, he succumbed to my request and agreed to arrange this for me, so that I could at least have a CT scan carried out at the hospital. I felt somewhat relieved at this point but also a bit nervous as well.

Around this same time, I had decided to travel to Coffs Harbour in New South Wales for a few days with some friends to watch the World Rally Championship.

Early one morning in September 2014 as we drove into Coffs Harbour in New South Wales, on our way to watch some of the WRC stages I received a phone call on my mobile phone. The call was from the Medical Imaging Department of the hospital in Brisbane. The lady calling informed me that a CT scan procedure had been arranged for the following week and upon my return from the WRC, I attended this appointment as scheduled, to have the scan that I had earlier requested, carried out.

One week later I was called back into the hospital again to receive the results of the scan. At this meeting the specialist said to me "We have noticed something strange in your CT scan report. There appears to be a lump sitting below your navel. Have you noticed anything different recently?" I replied, "No I haven't, and why do you ask me that?"

He said, "Let me see if I can find it." He then proceeded to massage my lower stomach and then said, "Oh yes, there is a hard lump there which seems to be about the size of a pea, here you feel it yourself?" I placed my fingers under my navel and yes, I could feel it at the same place.

He then suggested that it might be best to have a needle biopsy carried out to see what it really was. I agreed to this, expecting that he might carry it out there and then in his office, but he said "No, it needs to be carried out under an Ultrasound procedure."

"I will arrange for you to have an Ultrasound Guided Needle Biopsy procedure here next week, in the Medical Imaging Department of the hospital."

I agreed again to have this biopsy carried out and I returned to the hospital the following week and I had the needle inserted into my stomach. I will never forget the clicking noise of the needle biopsy insertion and then the cut to remove part of the suspicious lump. It sounded exactly like a handgun being cocked before being fired.

A week later the biopsy results had been completed and returned to the cancer department, from the hospital Pathology laboratory. I went once again into the office fearing what the outcome might be this time around, but I was most certainly not prepared for the shock that I was just about to receive.

The specialist said, "Please take a seat and sit down, I have now received your biopsy results from the Pathology Department and it's both good news and bad news for you." I said, "I will have both of them please, if you don't mind." He then replied, "Well, it looks like your Non-Hodgkin's Lymphoma is ok as there is 'nothing' showing up in the report, but the lump that we discovered is what we call a Metastatic Melanoma."

I said "How on earth could I have melanoma? I have never had a skin wart, tag, lesion, I don't get sunburnt, I don't lie on the beach, I wear a hat, I don't use suntan beds.

That doesn't make any sense and what does Metastatic mean?" He said, "It means that the cancer has started somewhere else in your body, at what we refer to as being a primary point, and it has then managed to spread throughout your entire body at this stage." I was in total disbelief and shock once again. I said, "What happens now from here on?" He replied that this type of Melanoma cancer wasn't his speciality, but he would arrange for me to see a melanoma specialist at the hospital as soon as possible. A week later I had another appointment with a melanoma specialist who informed me that the only real way forward to proceed with this latest situation would be for me to have a whole-body PET scan carried out, to see just how bad things might be. I was then referred for a hospital PET scan the following week. At this stage now I was totally petrified with what the outcome might be. I don't think I slept for the entire week. When the day came for the result to be announced it was totally catastrophic. I was called into the office where I took a seat, only to be delivered a shocking result.

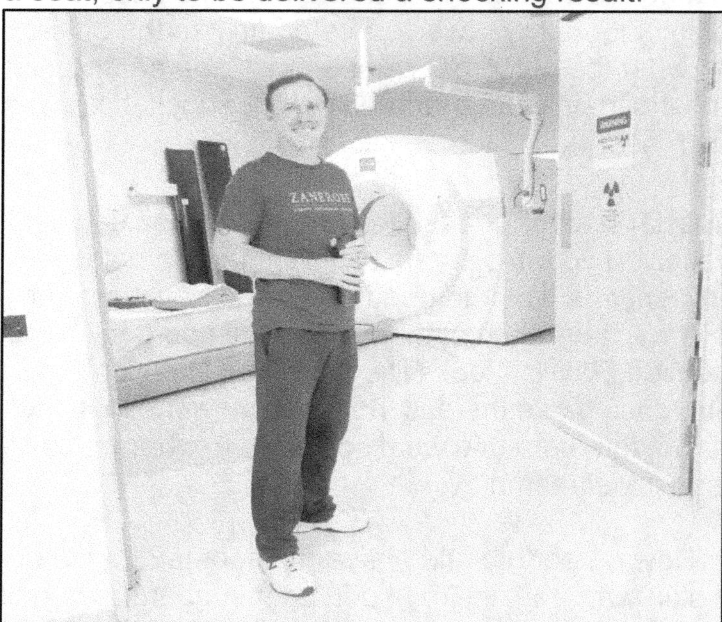

The CT scan which found the first Tumour

I was told that the scan had been unable to locate any primary cancer anywhere in my body and that was because the cancer unfortunately had now metastasised throughout my entire body. It had spread everywhere, except to my brain at this point. I was riddled with cancer.

I then asked what options were there left for me now, if any, only to be told we think at the most you have only 'three months left to live' and you might just make it to Christmas if you're very lucky and now might be a good time while you still can, to get all your affairs into some sort of order.

I asked if there were any new treatments available that I might be able to try and I was told that there were some new targeted therapies which had just been introduced and which were currently on clinical trials at that time. I said, "Surely I can try something if you think that I only have three months left to live now at the most?"

Before I left the hospital, I was given a script to collect some medication from the hospital pharmacy and an additional script for more medication to be collected again at the hospital the following week.

I was placed on these trial drugs which were known as Tafinlar and Mekinist. There were no expectations as to how they might work for me, but it was most certainly worth a try. I was told that the treatment mainly worked with patients that had a BRAF V600E mutation, however as mine was a BRAF V600K mutation there was a chance that they might still work for me as well. These drugs are part of what is known as a targeted therapy treatment which is primarily designed to remove the protective layer which the cancer cells are known to use, in order to protect themselves from being attacked by the body's own immune system.

As my body's immune system had already been destroyed by the unnecessary chemotherapy in 2011, I wasn't sure if this would work for me, but I had no other options left now at this stage but to try it. Since being told this latest diagnosis just the week before, I had already tried to access a new clinical trial which was going on called EBC46. The trial was being conducted at the Princess Alexandra hospital in Brisbane. However, since my cancer was classified as being too severe and advanced, that regrettably, I could not be admitted onto the trial. This EBC46 treatment was being developed from berries that grew on the Blushwood trees, in the Atherton Tablelands region of North Queensland. It had been found to work successfully on animals including the Tasmanian Devils, who had developed cancerous tumours on their faces. The tests had shown that when the cancer tumours appeared on the devils faces, they were then injected with an EBC46 treatment, which within days would then dry out to form a scab, which later dropped off. I did manage to buy this drug later in a syrup substance from the United States, but unfortunately it didn't show up as having any effect on my melanoma whatsoever. Again once, I had certainly tried.

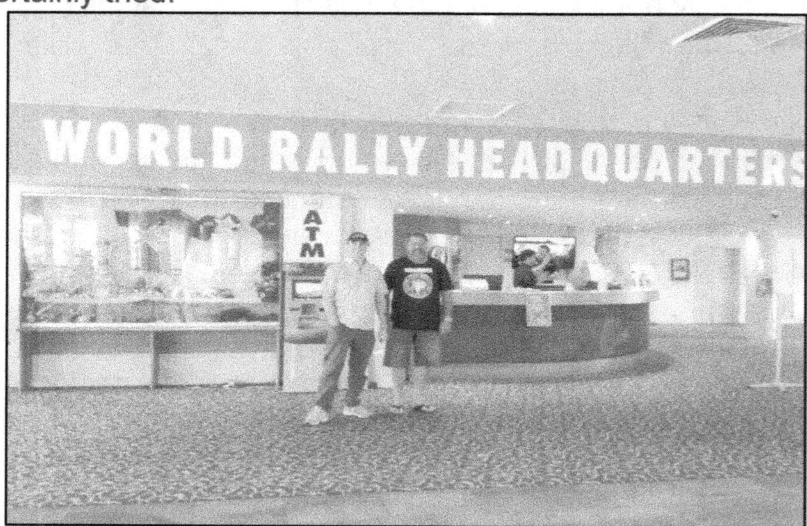

Robin and Whitey at the World Rally Coffs Harbour 2014

ALMOST THE END

I commenced the Tafinlar and Mekinist targeted therapy treatment in early October 2014 and I continued taking it daily. One day in early December as I was driving back home from the Gold Coast in Queensland, I suddenly started to develop severe sweats, chills and uncontrollable shaking. I pulled over to the side of the road and stopped for a moment, however the symptoms continued. I eventually managed to keep driving and stopping regularly until I finally made it home, where I then went straight to bed.

This scenario was to continue like this for the next five days until finally my wife told me that I really needed to go to the hospital for help.

Eventually I agreed to this, and we drove straight to the Emergency Department of a hospital in Brisbane where I had been attending at this time. After the usual waiting time in the Emergency Department, I was eventually taken to a cubicle where I was placed on a series of intravenous saline drips for several hours and the staff said I appeared to be comfortable at this stage. Around 11.00pm that same evening, which was around eight hours after I had been admitted earlier, my family left the hospital to return to our home in Burpengary, where we were living at this time. A short time later after they had left the ward, I was visited by an emergency doctor from the department. After he had carried out a quick check of me, he then looked into my eyes and immediately reached out above my bed and hit the Emergency Alarm button.

The next thing I remember was my bed being rushed out of the ward by the very same doctor, with a group of nurses helping him to push it straight down the hospital corridor and into the Cardiac Resuscitation theatre.

The theatre doors were pushed wide open by hitting them with the hospital bed frame as I was pushed in.

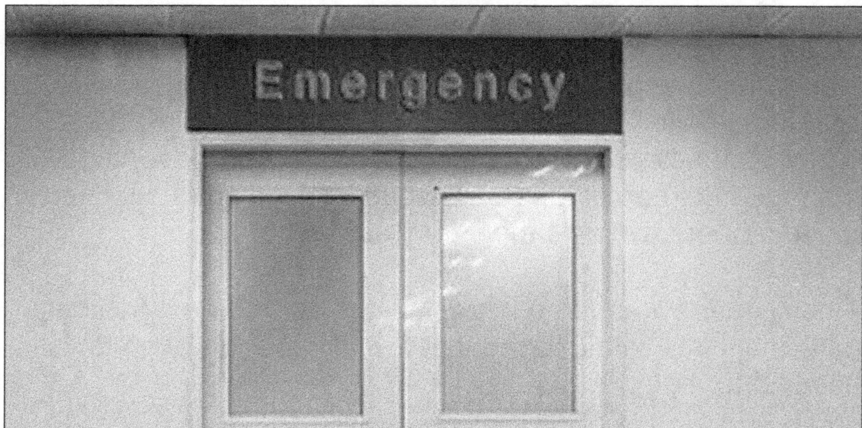

Cardiac Resuss Emergency Doors December 2014

I didn't realise then that I was in a very bad way. My family were telephoned at home around 12.30am to inform them of the immediate emergency situation that was unfolding at the hospital and could they please try to get back again as quickly as possible, as I was deteriorating very rapidly and I might have to be placed onto a life support machine, in an attempt to keep me alive and they needed the family's permission for them to be able to do this.

My family were totally shocked to receive this call, as when they had left me earlier in the evening, I appeared to be comfortable and doing okay from the nurse's report.

We had never discussed this type of thing before and we had nothing in place, nor had we agreed to anything previously, regarding my wishes for any life support equipment.

They rushed straight back to the hospital, picking up a speeding fine along the way and parked straight outside the hospital entrance doors. By this stage I had already been fitted with approximately sixteen different intravenous tubes inserted in various positions throughout my entire body.

My arms were full of drips, as well as all sorts of monitors on my chest. My neck had been cut open in various places and I could feel the warm blood oozing everywhere around my throat with almost a feeling like my throat had just been slashed wide open with a razor blade. I then had a tube inserted into my bladder and at the same time I had several intravenous tubes pushed up through the arteries in both my legs, directly towards my heart.

These were the most painful lines and the most difficult of them all, due to the fact that as they tried to push these intravenous lines up through my arteries, I kept sliding away from them along the leather mattress on the bed frame and two of the theatre nurses had to physically pull each of my arms towards them on both sides of the bed, so that the doctors could push the lines up through the arteries in both legs and directly towards my heart.

This was in addition to all the other tubes that were already running directly from my neck to my heart. I only found out later that these tubes, from where my neck was cut open hadn't reached to my heart after all. I knew at this point that I was in a very bad way, and I feared the worst. I prayed to God that he would help me survive this suffering, as it was so severe that I didn't think that I could possibly survive it for very much longer.

I was being given all sorts of drips from various intravenous bags, that were hanging everywhere around me at this stage. My family were allowed to enter the theatre room briefly to see me and they were all advised that my chances of survival at this stage were very slim indeed, if any at all.

My wife, my two sons and several of their friends who I also knew well, were all standing around me in the theatre bed. My bed was also surrounded by doctors and theatre nurses, and I think I can remember almost ten nurses and various doctors all looking down at me, at one stage.

My wife was able to ask me my wishes regarding life support and I said "No, just let me go, I don't want to be put onto any machines please, if it's time for me to go, then just let it happen."

After around six hours in the operating theatre, the South African emergency doctor, who had been at the forefront of this whole operation approached my family who were now sitting outside in the waiting area adjacent to the operating theatre doors.

The doctor told them that once the main adrenaline feed supply to my body had been removed, then I would either be able to continue to survive on my own behalf or else I would most likely have to be switched over onto a life support machine and that is where I would then remain. He wanted to know what my family's wishes would be at this time. None of my family knew what to do at this stage as it was such a shock that they were being asked to make such a very serious life or death decision immediately, considering that we had never discussed anything like this before at any time.

My wife at this point also remembered that whilst all this commotion was going on, her car was still parked outside the doors of the hospital Emergency Department.

She decided then that she would have to go back downstairs to the hospital emergency doors and move it, in case it could be blocking emergency vehicles access to the hospital. She left to move her car and whilst doing this she decided that, during all this mayhem to call her friend Ashana, to tell her what was happening with me.

She told her about what the doctor had just said regarding removing the adrenaline line, and that if I didn't manage to survive after this came out, then they needed to know whether to try to keep me alive by switching me on to a life support machine, or to just let me go. Her friend told her that around 6.30am I would make my own decision as to whether I wanted to continue to fight this awful disease or else I would just die. All this time I was still praying that the good Lord would stand with me and help me through this massive turbulence that was devastating my body.

I remained totally conscious the whole time that this was happening all around me and I never wish to be in that situation ever again. It was a terrible struggle and one that I will never forget, and I wouldn't wish it to happen to anyone else in their lifetime.

My family told the theatre doctor that I would make my own decision at that time as to whether I would continue to live or whether I would die. The nurses then removed the adrenaline infusion tube from my body at 6.15am and I remained fully conscious as I was being transferred at this stage across the corridor to the Intensive Care unit, directly opposite the operating theatre.

I was still in a very dangerous condition at this time, but I had managed to remain alive even thought I was still surrounded, by a mass of intravenous drips hanging out of every part of my body.

It was in this Intensive Care unit that I was to remain for the next two days before I was eventually transferred to a normal ward of the hospital. I had managed to survive this terrible onslaught and I was very grateful to the good Lord who had helped the doctors, nurses and my own family, to keep me alive during this whole ordeal.

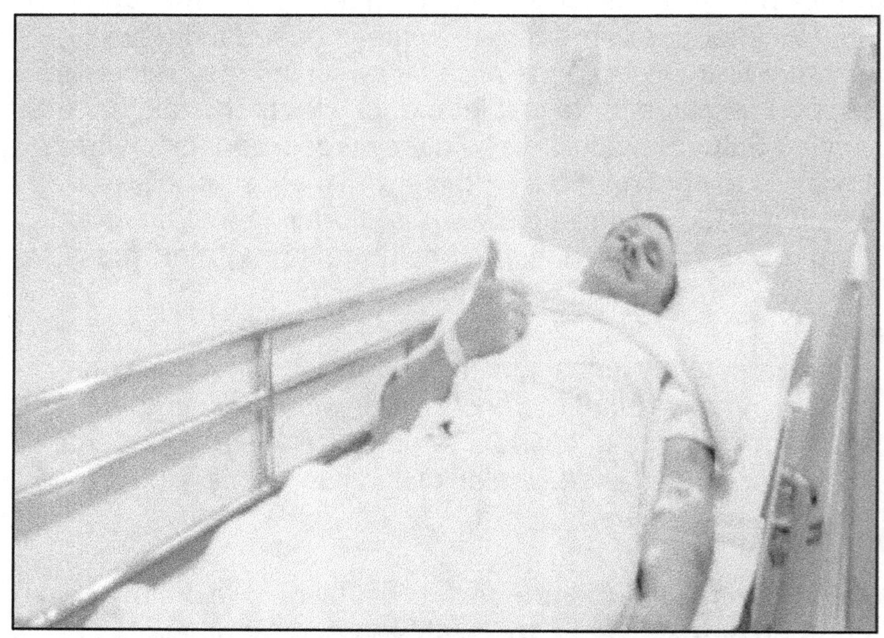

Robin in Intensive Care December 2014

I was finally able to return, back home once again a few days later and it had appeared from the pathology report which had now been completed, that at the time this had occurred, it was the medication that I had been receiving, which had triggered what is known as SIRS, which is an abbreviation for a condition known as Severe Immune Response Syndrome. I had indeed been very lucky to have survived this life-threatening situation.

I was advised to immediately stop taking the recommended daily dose of Tafinlar and Mekinist medication until my body had made a full recovery and returned to some sort of normality, after such a serious near-death experience.

I recommenced the trial medication once again after the Christmas period, albeit very nervously as I had now managed to make it past the three-month life expectancy period, and I was very thankful for it.

A few months later in April 2015 my son was passing out into the Australian Army at the Wagga Wagga military base situated in New South Wales. On the morning of our planned flight from Brisbane to Wagga Wagga, I suddenly developed the exact same symptoms again, that I had experienced in early December. I started shaking uncontrollably and I had the severe sweats and chills appear once again. I recognised these symptoms immediately from my previous episode and I was now forced to make a very difficult decision. Should I continue in my current condition, or should I cancel the trip and during all this, not see my own son's passing out parade? I made my own decision to stop the medication immediately and to go ahead with the planned trip. It was a very scary situation but again it appeared to me to be the right decision to make at this time.

I travelled to Brisbane where I then caught a flight to Wagga Wagga in New South Wales. After watching my sons passing out parade, I flew straight back home again to Brisbane the next day.

I commenced the treatment again within the next few days. Around two weeks later I was back at the hospital once again for my regular monthly appointment and I informed the oncologist of my recent circumstances and of what had just happened.

I how told her how I had decided to handle the situation myself, and that it had worked once again in my favour after stopping the treatment for just a few days.

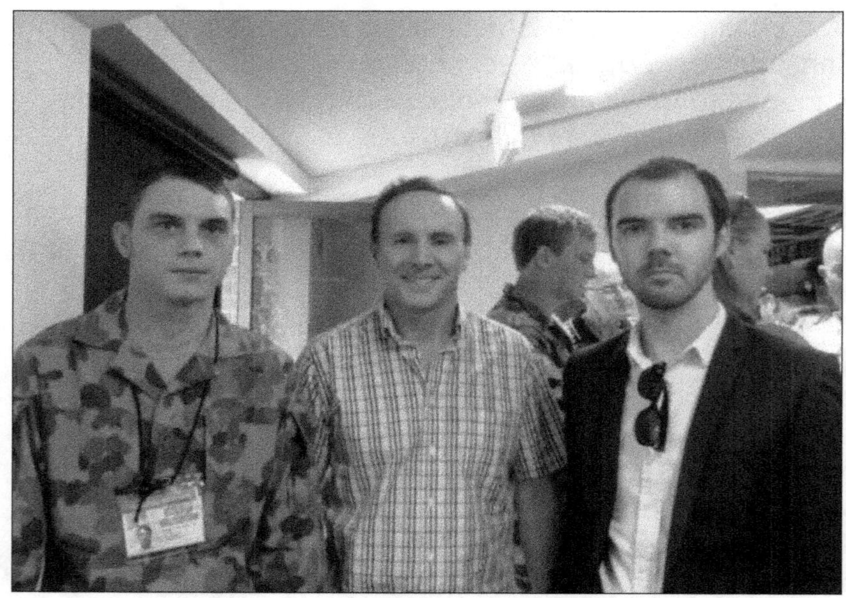

Robin and Andrew attending Philip's Army recruitment in 2015

The oncologist was shocked and told me that I should have come straight to the hospital. Nevertheless, I had survived another close call by making my own decision. I continued with this treatment until August 2015 when I had my next scheduled whole body PET scan.

This was to see what effect, if any, that this medication was having on my cancer, as I was now eight months past the life expectancy time frame I had been given in October 2014.

I was amazed to discover, that at this point I had achieved what is called a complete metabolic response or what is more commonly referred to in medical terms as being NED (this stands for No Evidence of Disease being found in the body at that time).

This meant that the cancer which I had been told would probably take my life within three months in October 2014, was now almost all gone. I had an amazing feeling of euphoria at this result. It was incredible and I was very thankful to everyone who had supported me on this journey so far. I had also continued to carry out my own research on this new treatment and I had discovered that at some point in the future the cancer would once again outsmart this combination therapy.

The targeted treatment worked in a similar way to approaching a barricade. The cancer approaches the barricade, but it is unable to get past the barrier. It then makes a retreat and has a rethink about how it might make it past this barricade again using a different type of approach. It decides to return once again, but this time the cancer cells decide to try getting around the 'right' hand side of the barricade. As before, the cancer cells fail in this approach once again. This process with some patients can continue for several years.

In other patients, it may only last just a few months, before the cancer regroups and launches a further onslaught once more.

What the cancer then does is to rethink its strategy at that point. Well, okay, we have tried to get straight through that barricade but that didn't work, we tried going around the right-hand side and that didn't work either, so we might just try to get around the left-hand side of the barricade.

Once this attempt is made and it succeeds, then the cancer is winning again as it has now managed to outsmart the treatment 'barricade' and it's on its way once more. This is also like sleeping medication. With continuous use each night, eventually the body starts to reject the medication and it ceases to work.

I knew that once this happened, I would have to have a Plan B ready to take effect, if I was to have any chance of continuing to survive the onslaught on my body a second time around.

In March 2016 it was arranged for me to have another whole-body PET scan carried out. The result of this scan continued to show that the cancer was still under some form of control at this time, which to me was a great outcome.

Unfortunately, a short time later due to an unexpected accident occurring, my health was impaired once again. I had accidently fallen several metres down off a mezzanine floor in my workshop and I had landed straight onto a concrete surface below on my lower back. As a result of this accident, I now had a broken pelvis to deal with as well.

This injury took several months of weekly rehabilitation at the Redcliffe hospital as I was unable to move around without using the aid of a pair of crutches.

All during this period, from my original diagnosis in September 2014 until March 2016, I had also been flying each month from Brisbane to Sydney and then travelling an hour each way in a taxi to Gladesville in the western suburbs of Sydney to attend a Chinese Acupuncture and Herbal remedies specialist, to try to help me rebuild my body's immune system, which had been totally destroyed after the previous five months of unnecessary chemotherapy.

I continued this herbal treatment for a further two years at cost of forty-two thousand dollars, until I was no longer able to afford it. In January 2017 I read about a vitamin medication called Laetrile (Amygladin) or B17, which it is more commonly referred to as, and how it was being widely used throughout various hospitals in Mexico for cancer.

This treatment was being used instead of regular chemotherapy. It was being manufactured from apricot kernels and it was also being administered to patients through various protocols, ranging from intravenous infusions to tablet forms.

I decided to try the tablet form and I had this sent each month to Australia, which I then took as a daily supplement medication.

Once again, unfortunately after around twelve months of taking this vitamin, I didn't appear to be having any success with it and it was only much later after further research that I discovered, that the medication had to be taken in conjunction with a particular enzyme, which I wasn't aware of at the time, for it to work effectively at destroying the cancer cells.

I had a further PET scan carried out at the hospital in Brisbane several months later.

Sadly, this uncovered that the cancer had now returned once again but this time it had now managed to crossover what is known as the body's blood/brain barrier, and it had been able to spread itself further, by entering my brain.

I was once again totally devastated, especially after I had been showing so much success up to this point, but at least I had managed to achieve twenty-four months longer in a survival stage than I had originally been expected to live. The question now was, what should I do from here? What options are there available to me now?

I requested a brain scan but this was not available to me so I contacted my own GP who suggested that I should arrange and pay for my own brain MRI scan, at a local medical imaging practice at Currimundi, on the Sunshine Coast in Queensland.

I booked the scan and paid around one thousand dollars to have this carried out. The results confirmed that, yes, I now had three brain tumours which were in keeping with what they referred to as intra-cerebral Metastatic Melanoma. This was further proof that the cancer had indeed managed to spread itself and I was now in a very precarious position.

The worst that I had been in for some time as the cancer had now managed to cross over the brain/blood barrier and had entered various parts of my brain.

During this time, I continued to carry out my daily research and I had been following a new Melanoma treatment which had recently been launched in the United States. It was an immunotherapy treatment designed to help retrain your body's own immune system into fighting the cancer cells.

An ex-Lord Mayor of Melbourne, and a man who had been instrumental in having the Australian Grand Prix relocated from Adelaide in South Australia to Melbourne in Victoria had recently been diagnosed with melanoma cancer that had also spread into his brain. This individual was a close friend of Hilary Clinton in the United States and in an approach, to enable him to be able to continue to spend more precious time with his grandchildren, he requested if he could be accepted onto a trial in the United States.

His request was successful, and he started the treatment, and soon later discovered that he had found success with it.

Upon his return to Australia, he decided to contact the then Australian Prime Minister Tony Abbot, whom he was closely acquainted with regarding having this treatment brought to Australia and being made available to patients who were in a similar situation to his own. The treatment was known as Keytruda or (Pembrolizumab), which was an immunotherapy treatment.

I discussed my latest research of this new immunotherapy treatment with the oncologist who I was still attending at the hospital in Brisbane at this time. I requested if I could please be offered it, as I knew that it had just been recently approved for use with melanoma patients in Australia. Instead, I was offered a different treatment, which was a combination of two other drugs.

One was called Opdivo (Nivolumab) and the other one was called Yervoy (Ippillumab) or 'Ippy' as it is more commonly referred to.

I had read up on this combination treatment earlier and I felt very uncomfortable with it, as the side effects that patients had been experiencing from it were huge.

I was told that this treatment would be better suited for me instead of receiving the Keytruda (Pembrolizumab). I was still unsure about this but knowing that I now needed to commence some other form of treatment urgently, if I was to continue my fight to survive, I agreed to have it. I left the hospital with a plan to return once again in two weeks' time to commence this new treatment. A few days later I was still feeling very uncomfortable with my own decision to accept this new treatment.

I decided then to contact the oncologist at the hospital to inform them that I wanted to change my mind and that I no longer wished to commence this combination therapy of Opdivo and Yervoy. I knew that the Opdivo was a similar drug to the Keytruda and that the only real difference between the two immunotherapy treatments was that they were being manufactured by two different pharmaceutical companies. I told the oncologist that I would still prefer to be treated with the new Keytruda immunotherapy treatment instead.

This was the drug that I had already been researching for some time. My request was agreed to, and I started the first treatment of Keytruda immunotherapy in February 2017.

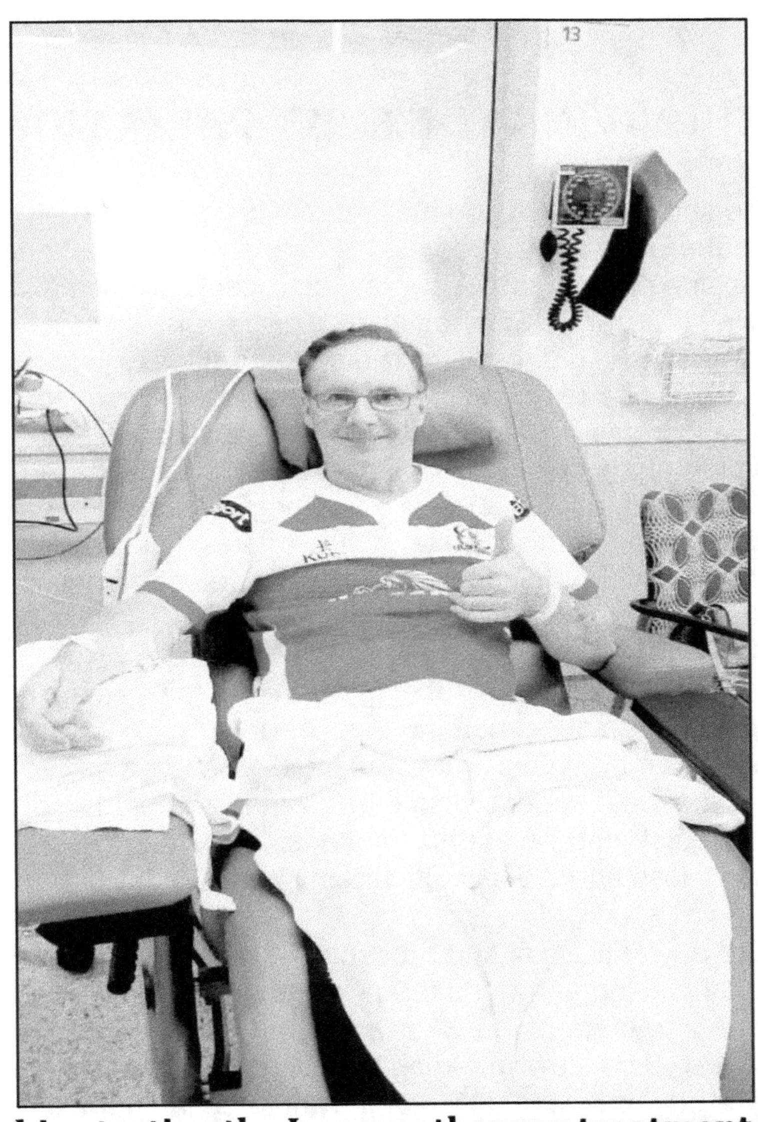

Robin starting the Immunotherapy treatment he selected for himself in 2017

SURVIVING THE FIRST RADIATION

At the same time as I commenced my chosen treatment, I was referred to a brain radiologist at another hospital on the south side of Brisbane, regarding a procedure which is known as Gamma Knife radiation. This is where a steel frame is screwed directly into your skull, which is then bolted onto a sliding trolley frame. This frame is then pushed inside a radiation machine and each tumour is individually targeted with pin-point precision to provide accurate radiation strikes. This is opposite to using whole brain radiation, which can produce very serious long term side effects. It is a very precise form of radiation treatment, directed straight into the centre of the cancer tumour to destroy it.

I had already studied the effects of whole brain radiation and I decided this was something that I certainly didn't want to have carried out. One lady I contacted in Victoria had already lost her speech from it and various others I had contacted shared similar horror stories, including severe memory loss and the loss of certain nerves.

On the day of the planned procedure, I travelled to the hospital arriving at around 6.00am in the morning. I had left home an hour earlier, as I knew the early morning peak hour traffic would be slowly starting to build up as usual coming into the city and I certainly didn't want to be late for this important appointment. As I waited outside in the designated patient area, I started chatting with other patients who were also starting to arrive, to have the exact same procedure carried out, that I was going to have.

We were all very nervous at this point, obviously concerned about what was going to be ahead of us that day. One young lady that I spoke with, had flown to Brisbane from Townsville in North Queensland, leaving her small children to be cared for by her parents.

It was a long trip on her own I thought, and then to have this procedure carried out as well, so I decided to share with her some of the research that I had already conducted and why I felt, that it was much safer to have this Gamma Knife radiation procedure carried out, rather than having whole brain radiation. Once the doors of the building opened then we all entered together, wishing each other good luck for our respective operations. Everyone was placed into their various cubicles to change into surgical gowns, which we would then all be wearing during the various procedures that day.

I was then put onto a hospital bed before being transferred to the Medical Imaging Department of the hospital, as apparently the brain radiologist, who would be carrying out the procedure required more recent up-to-date scans to confirm his accuracy of each target. This was very important so that he would have all the very latest information on any new tumour developments and the various locations of the tumours inside my brain. This would then assist him to be able to pin-point those areas where he needed to target the laser radiation treatment effectively to destroy the tumours.

After the brain scan was completed, I was transferred back to the Gamma Knife radiation team, to await the results of the scan. This again became a very anxious waiting time. Around an hour later the brain radiation specialist came back to see me in the waiting area.

I felt genuine warmth towards this doctor straight away and I had a feeling of trust that sadly I had never had before, due to all the negligence I had previously suffered. He said to me. "I'm very sorry to have to tell you that instead of the original three brain tumours that showed up in your last scan, there are now seven tumours in your brain, in total. I have never treated seven tumours before at the very same time, but I will do my very best for you."

I was totally devastated again in the knowledge that instead of facing a procedure, on an expected three brain tumours, that I was now facing more serious radiation on seven tumours, which was going to be very difficult to survive, if that was at all possible. At this point I replied. "You can only do your best and I'm very confident that you will be successful." I also knew at this stage there were only three people that I could ask to help me through what I was about to experience in my brain and that was my faith in God, my radiation specialist, and myself.

I prayed that God would guide him with his work, to successfully help me through this procedure, which I knew was going to be very severe for me to survive.

I was then pushed deep inside the radiation machine and that is where I was to remain fully conscious for the entire duration of the two-hour procedure. Each of the brain tumours was struck individually with the radiation device. I could feel the sensation happening as the laser penetrated through my skull on each strike.

It was a very frightening experience and certainly one that I never had expected I would have to endure in my lifetime. I lay in the machine feeling the pulse of each strike and I prayed that each strike would be successful in striking into the centre of each tumour and destroy it.

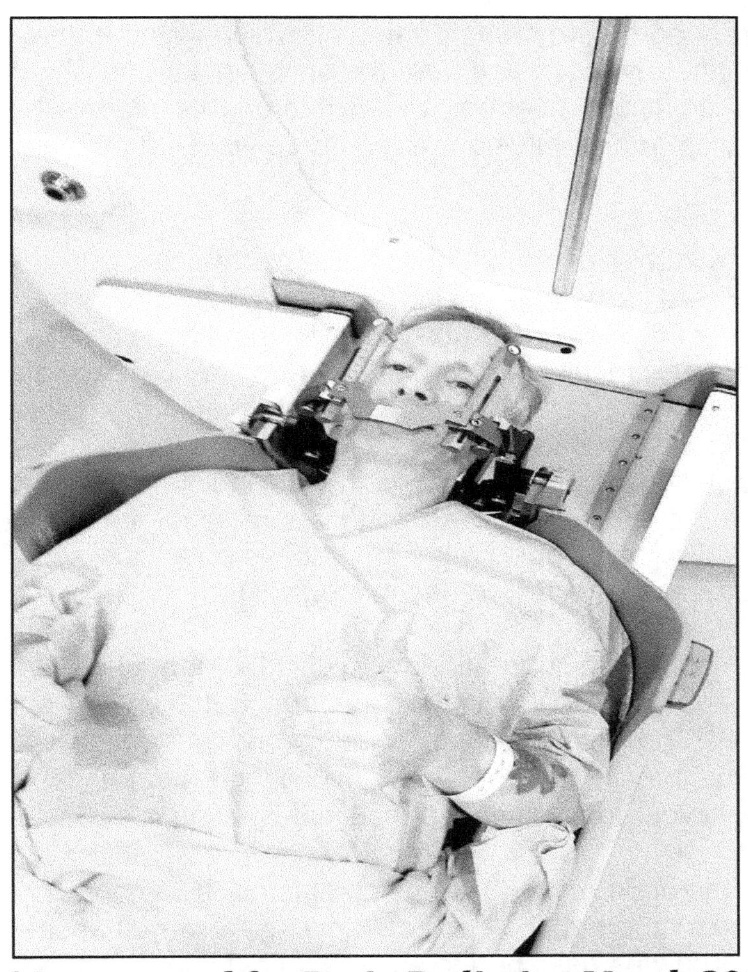

Robin prepared for Brain Radiation March 2017

It certainly felt like it had been an eternity and it was such a relief towards the end when I finally heard the voice speaking to me from inside the radiation machine telling me, "It's all over now, you have done very well, and we will bring you out of the machine in a few minutes time." I returned to the waiting area once again and undressed out of the hospital gown I was still wearing, and I switched back into my own clothes before travelling back home.

I continued the Keytruda treatment, which was the treatment I had already requested from the oncologist before the initial brain radiation procedure. I remained on this treatment receiving regular infusions every three weeks for several months.

On the 29th of June 2017 I had another brain scan completed at the hospital in Brisbane. This was to check the results of the Gamma Knife radiation that I had carried out in March. The results showed that there were no new brain tumours and that the previous tumours that had previously been radiated, were already actually shrinking and so was the swelling inside my brain. It was obvious, that after having seven brain tumours struck with laser radiation throughout my skull, that it would cause me to develop a lot of swelling, or oedema as it's referred to in medical terms.

Overall, this was a great result to discover that I had not developed any new brain tumours during this period, and I was also now starting to feel more confident that the original treatment that I had chosen for myself was indeed working in my favour to produce the results in fighting my cancer.

After the brain procedure was completed, I was prescribed a steroid by the radiation doctor know as Dexamethasone. This drug was designed to assist with helping to reduce the swelling inside my brain caused by the huge amount of radiation procedures.

The downside of this drug was that it caused severe sleep insomnia and I was really struggling to try to get any sleep each night. I had also discovered through fresh research regarding a plant called Indian Frankincense, which is known from the three wise men in the Bible and how it could also help to reduce the swelling (oedema in my brain).

The one that I selected was known as Boswellia Serrata. This was available in a capsule, and it was extracted from the resin gum of the Boswellia shrubs that grew in mountainous terrain in India. It was a very difficult plant to harvest, as the local people had to climb the mountains to extract the bark, which was also eaten by wild goats.

I continued the Dexamethasone which I was prescribed for a few more months, however the insomnia was becoming so severe that I later switched over to using the Boswellia instead, which I found helped me significantly and reduced my headaches and enabled me to start sleeping again.

The following month in July 2017 I was asked to undertake a further whole-body PET scan at the hospital in Brisbane. The concept behind having these PET scans is that the body is infused with a supply of glucose (sugar) through a cannula needle inserted into either arm, after which you are then left to rest in a room for an hour whilst the glucose is then distributed around the body, through your own blood supply vessels.

As cancer is well known to feed from the glucose/sugar inside the body, the resulting scan then shows this up in the images, to identify where the cancer is feeding from this glucose in the body. It is referred to in the medical world as being 'uptakes' or feeding zones.

This scan showed there was no uptake in my brain at that time. However, there appeared to be two new areas of suspicious activity in my body.

This was rather concerning; however, I was told at the time that these could simply have just been areas of inflammation or old previous scar tissue and further MRI scans should be considered for more accuracy.

I requested that I should still be given the chance to keep being treated with the Keytruda for longer, as it stated on the PET scan report that it 'could only' just be inflammation showing up instead of new tumours. Sadly, my request was refused by the treating oncologist at this time.

I had also decided a few months earlier that I wanted to avoid another combination treatment that had been offered to me, known as Opdivo (Nivolumab) and Yervoy (Ipillumab) or Ippy, as it was more commonly referred to.

This was due to the severe side effects that I had discovered could happen from it. I was also still very nervous from the terrible experience I had suffered previously in December 2014. I had read up where some people had died from this combination treatment and that the auto-immune conditions that it instigated could cause severe liver, kidney and colon damage such as colitis. I decided in July 2017 that now might be the right time for me to start looking into various alternative treatments that might be available overseas.

I started researching cancer clinics in Germany and Virotherapy in Latvia. I had also researched RGCC laboratories in Greece. This is where a sample of a patient's own blood is sent for analysis, in order to test which treatment, they may or may not respond to and if it was possible to produce a vaccine from the results of these blood tests. In August 2017 I decided that I would travel to Germany to attend a cancer clinic located in Berlin. This clinic had been referred to me by a lady living in Western Australia who had attended it for her breast cancer. The cost of this treatment for the two weeks totalled fifty thousand dollars.

To enable me to fund this I sold a classic car that I had built earlier, and I withdrew further funding from my rapidly diminishing superannuation fund.

I contacted my family who live in Northern Ireland, and they offered to meet me in Berlin to support me with this treatment. My mother, my two sisters and my two brothers-in-law all attended with me. The Berlin clinic performed several different types of treatment during the two weeks I spent there, which unfortunately later showed that I had not managed to achieve any success from their treatments.

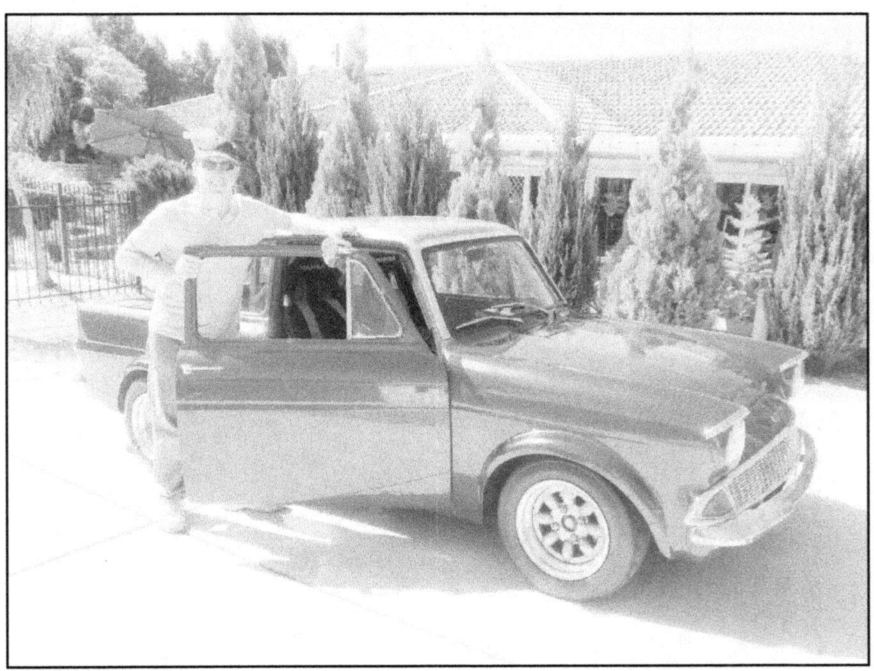

Robin with the Ford Anglia classic car he built and sold to fund his own treatment in Germany

I was given hyperthermia treatment, which is where you are placed inside an incubation chamber, which is then heated up until it reaches a maximum temperature and where you can no longer withstand the temperature inside it anymore.

My head remained outside of the chamber, and I was allowed to sip some water during this incubation period, but it was hampered for me, since even though the window in the clinic room was open for ventilation, there were people standing outside below the window of the building smoking, and the toxins flowed through into my incubation chamber.

I couldn't handle this any more than thirty minutes, as I was totally saturated in sweat and the enormous heat was giving me a terrible headache. I was then removed from the chamber and taken to another treatment room nearby.

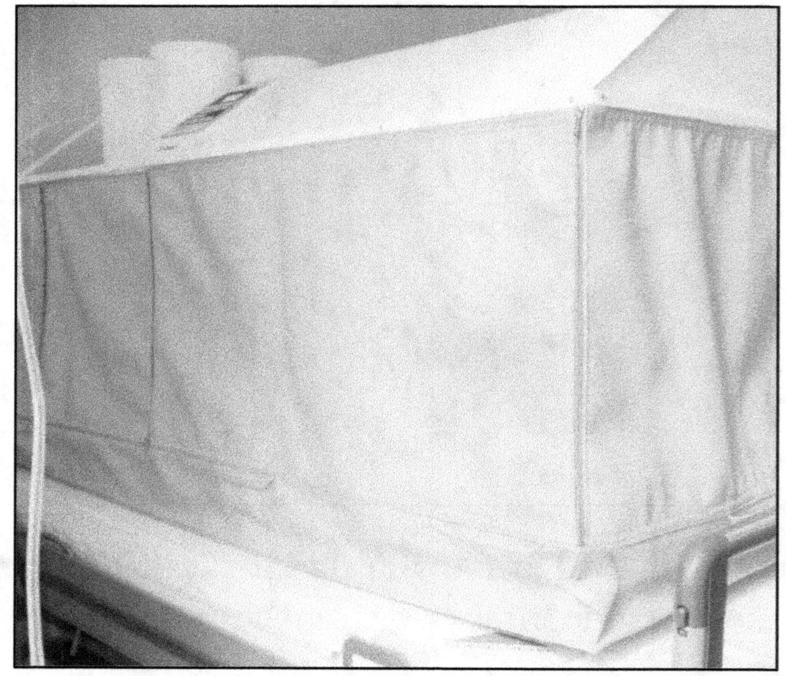

Hyperthermia Chamber in the Berlin Clinic 2017

In this room a tube was placed inside my colon and a colonic flush commenced via an automatic flushing machine. It was a very invasive treatment and extremely painful.

After this part of the treatment was completed, I was then infused with coffee enemas. This is a procedure where your colon is filled with coffee for approximately thirty minutes, whilst heat is applied to your liver using hot towels. It's known as a liver cleansing technique. After this you are then transferred to a different room again, where you are given oxygen therapy. This is where a portion of your blood is removed via a cannula needle inserted into your arm. The removed blood is then pumped through an oxygen machine, before it is returned into your body once again.

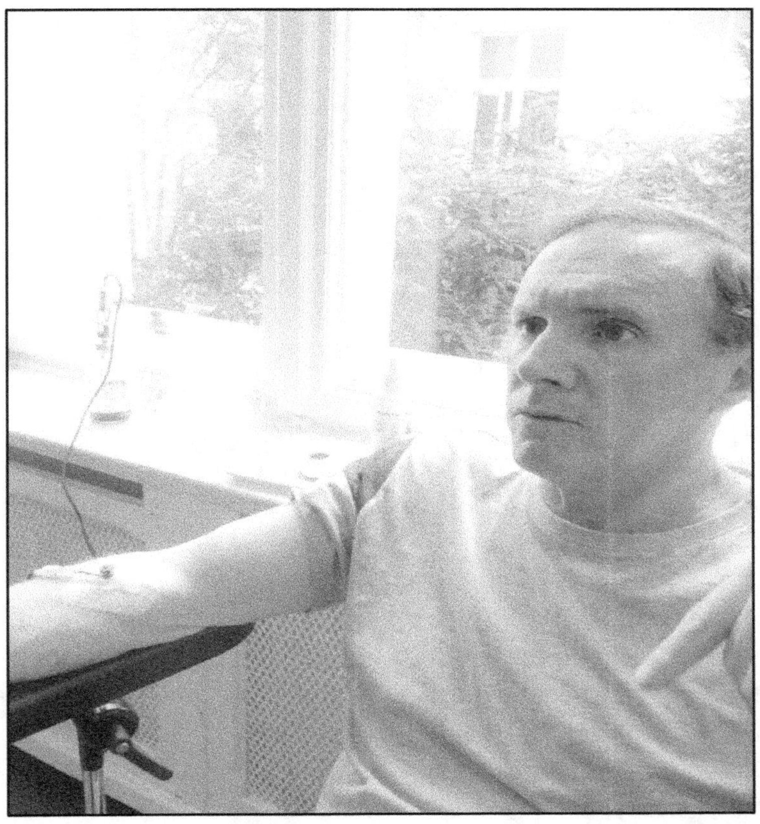

Robin receiving Oxygen Blood Therapy in Berlin August 2017

This is very similar to a procedure used in some bicycle marathons, such as the Tour de France and it's really a form of illegal doping. The young male nurse in the clinic told me that both he and his brother, who competed regularly in long distance bicycle race events, had tested this personally on each other and it had been shown to work, by comparing their various race result times.

Other treatments involved the arm and leg muscles being placed under extreme heat pressure presses to try to kill the cancer cells inside them, that I was told had appeared on the last scans, but I wasn't convinced that this was indeed correct information.

I also received mistletoe extract infusions which are known in Germany as Helixor, and where it is used instead of giving chemotherapy. I purchased several months' supply of this mistletoe extract (Helixor) treatment, whilst I was in Germany using a script that the German doctor had provided me with and I brought it back home with me to Australia, where I started to use it for my weekly infusions.

It was an extremely tough two weeks and the melanoma vaccine Rigvir that I wished to try from Riga, the capital of Latvia (Rigvir, which stood for Riga Virus) arrived whilst I was attending the clinic.

I had several days of constant intravenous infusions and various types of injections carried out. Blood tests were taken, both before and after the treatments were completed. Sadly, none of these treatments had shown any positive results. The best part of the trip to Berlin was catching up with my family, whom I hadn't seen for several years.

Before leaving Germany, I purchased additional vials of Rigvir injections.

I brought these back to Australia packed inside dry ice and sealed in a large saucepan, which I then placed inside a moulded plastic suitcase I had purchased earlier in Berlin. The virus had to be maintained at a constant minus twenty degrees temperature, otherwise the treatment could be spoilt.

The cost of the six months' supply of Rigvir injections was one hundred thousand dollars, which devastated what was barely left in my superannuation account at this time.

As I had anticipated bringing this additional supply of Rigvir treatment back to Australia I had already purchased a special medical fridge to store it in, as a normal household fridge couldn't maintain, the lower temperature it required of minus twenty degrees.

This was the temperature that the treatment needed to protect itself with. Another issue that I had already prepared for was that in the event of a power outage the treatment could be 'spoilt' if the lower temperature was temporarily lost, and everything would then be defrosted.

To allow for the unexpected happening I had pre-purchased a battery backup system, which used two large marine batteries and other timing devices to operate it. This was very important, because if I was away from home for any given length of time and the power had been switched off and it came back on again later, I might not have known that it had been switched off in the first instance.

If this was to happen, then the treatment would have been destroyed in my absence, without me even being aware that this had happened. For several months I had continued to research the combination targeted therapy treatment once again.

This was the treatment which I had taken previously known as Tafinlar and Mekinist and the one that had already shown me some success, albeit only for a short period of fifteen months.

The study had shown that in the United States some patients had been re-trialled using the same drugs a second time around and were having renewed success with it.

Even though the cancer-free period was much shorter than the previous one, any cancer-free period in my own opinion was a good one.

I requested from the oncologist if it would be possible for me to trial this targeted therapy treatment again, a second time around, based on the recent research which I had already conducted. Sadly, I was told that no, it wouldn't work a second time around and that I didn't qualify for it again anyway as I had failed it the first time. I told the oncologist about my ongoing research and especially regarding the retrials, that were currently under way in the United States, but unfortunately it was to no avail.

Even today here in Australia, this treatment is now being supplied to hospital cancer patients a second time around with similar success, as the original research had initially confirmed. After I was refused this treatment again, later in September 2017 I was then offered the treatment which I had originally been most afraid of, as unfortunately there was nothing else available to me and I had now very sadly been taken off the Keytruda. I had been removed from the treatment on the pretext that it was no longer working for me. This was the treatment which I had originally selected for myself in the very first instance and now I had been taken off it. I was told that the only option left for me now would be to undergo six courses of Opdivo (Nivolumab) and Yervoy (Ipillumab).

I was very fearful of this combination treatment after having read up on the severe side effects it had been known to cause in numerous patients, but I had now been left with no other option at this stage and I desperately needed to try something, if I was to continue controlling the cancer and to stay alive. I was told that I would be given six cycles of the combination treatment of Opdivo and Yervoy.

At the end of the six cycles, I would be placed onto an Opdivo single agent treatment for maintenance purposes.

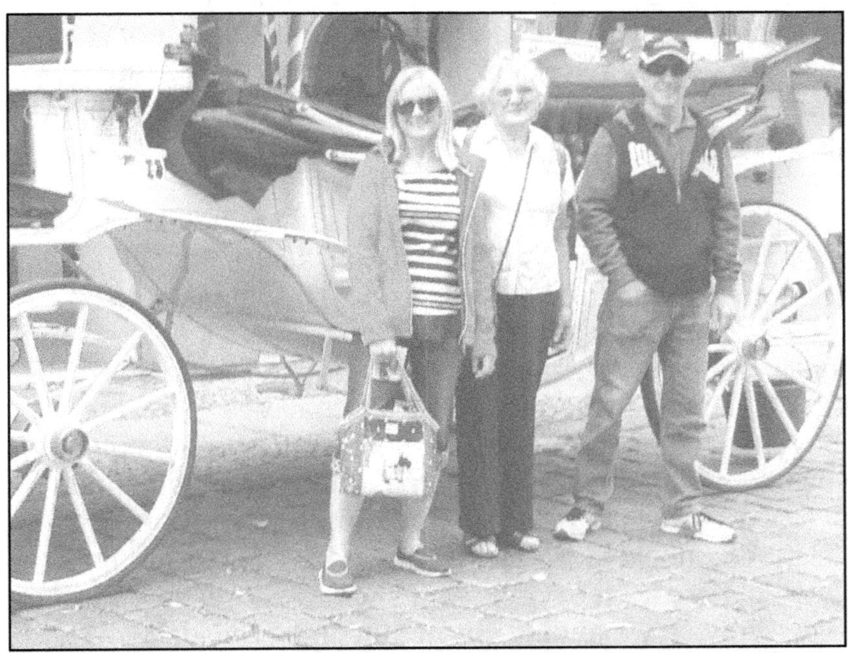

Robin, Mum and Sister Valerie in Berlin 2017

THE SECOND ONSLAUGHT

Before commencing any treatment, it is standard protocol for a patient to complete blood tests in advance. This is to ensure that the body's organs are normal and more to the point that it is safe to commence giving the treatment. I had already started to request my own blood test results from my own GP, prior to attending all my hospital appointments. Over the years I had also learnt to read and understand these blood tests, especially my liver and kidney enzymes. This way I could recognise in advance if anything didn't seem to be quite normal ahead of my scheduled appointments.

The date was arranged for the very first combination infusion of Opdivo and Yervoy. I had the usual customary appointment with the oncologist prior to going into the treatment rooms. I had already received my blood test results prior to attending this appointment from my own GP and I could clearly see that my liver enzymes were ten times above what their normal levels were. At this appointment I was told by the oncologist to proceed to the infusion rooms as they were waiting for me to commence my treatment. At this stage I decided it was time to speak up. I asked the oncologist if my blood test results are, okay? The oncologist said, "Oh yes, we should check that first, shouldn't we?" I said, "If you don't mind, please, that would be good."

After checking the results on a nearby desktop computer it became immediately apparent that my liver enzyme levels were not okay, but rather that they were indeed approximately ten times above their normal limits.

At this stage I was then told "Oh no, you can't have any treatment today, it's far too dangerous, we will have to leave it for a week and then we will get you to redo your blood tests again, to see if your liver has returned back to normal."

I was shocked at this. Should I not of asked this question and commenced the treatment, I fear to think what the outcome could have been. This is another example of, if you are ever in any doubt, then shout out for a second opinion to give yourself some peace of mind.

T.Bili	11	8	8	6	12	umol/L (2-20)
Alk.P	205	156	190	219	268	U/L (30-115)
GGT	373	175	167	176	173	U/L (0-70)
ALT	500	165	70	158	203	U/L (0-45)
AST	184	72	51	101	101	U/L (0-41)
LD	249	182	230	242	247	U/L (80-250)
Calcium	2.28	2.57	2.37	2.16	2.19	mmol/L (2.25-2.

Blood test results showing Liver ALT 500 when it should be between 0 - 45

I left the hospital and went to the nearest park with my wife. We were both shocked at what had just happened, and we sat down together at an adjacent park bench to discuss this latest finding. I decided to start using a herb, known as Sillybum Marianum (Milk Thistle) to help detoxify my liver, along with another herb called Artichoke. When I returned to the hospital two weeks later, my liver had restored itself back to acceptable levels, which would allow the treatment to commence and I told the oncologist what I had taken to get this result, but in their opinion, it must have just been a virus and it was gone now.

I have continued to take Sillybum (Milk Thistle) every day since then to help keep my liver enzymes under control, as immunotherapy is widely known to affect them. It was now time to proceed to the hospital treatment rooms to commence the first of the eight recommended treatment cycles. It was now late September 2017.

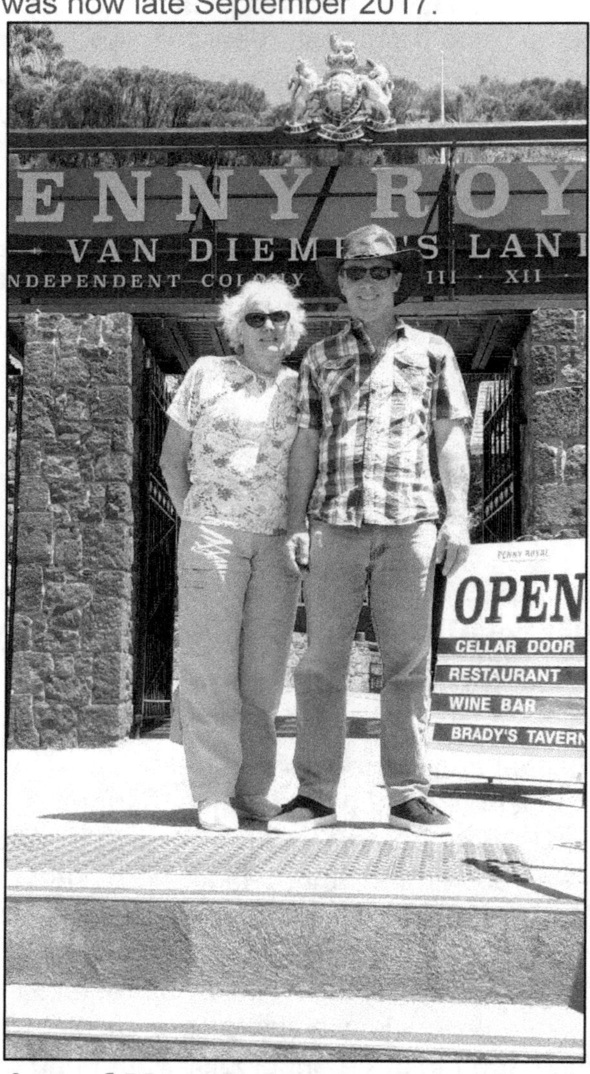

Robin and Mum in Launceston, Tasmania

Unfortunately, as I had already expected, I was only able to manage four of the scheduled eight cycles of this treatment. The reason that I only managed to have four treatment cycles was because I almost died from it. The treatment that I had feared the most from the very beginning had certainly shown its true potential. After the fourth cycle I became violently ill. One morning as I got up out of bed, I started to vomit so much that my stomach lining started to come out. I lay on the bedroom floor, and I was very quickly surrounded, by a pink coloured jelly-like substance, which I later discovered was my stomach lining coming out.

I spent the rest of the day shuffling around the house, carrying a plastic bucket with me, which was slowly filling up from the lining coming out from my stomach. At one stage as I lay on the ground, I asked the good Lord if he would take me, please, as I couldn't stand the pain and suffering any longer, of my stomach lining coming out.

This was to continue for several days until my wife drove me to the hospital Emergency Department, where I was to remain sitting for several hours practically dying, whilst people with a wooden splinter in their finger were taken before me. I couldn't even sit in a chair. Several times I walked over to where the hospital dirty laundry trolley was sitting and I removed all the old soiled, bed-linen sheets, just to try to make up a bed for myself on the floor, where I could lie down for a while, as I was so overcome with pain and exhaustion. This was usually enough to trigger an alarm and to have me taken to a hospital bed. This was to continue for a further six weeks, upon each return visit to the hospital. It was a horrendous time.

Over consecutive weeks, I would continue, to be in the hospital for days on end, receiving daily saline hydration infusions.

The treatment was continuing to leave me extremely dehydrated, despite drinking litres of water each day. The cannula would be removed and then replaced again the next day. One day the cannula hadn't been inserted properly into my vein. It was only pushed into the skin, and I knew that it wasn't correct. I was then given a Potassium infusion, as this was apparently what my body needed to be given at that time.

Over the next thirty minutes infusion period the stinging pain became so bad that my arm turned completely yellow and purple. I removed the cannula from my arm myself, much to the dismay of the hospital staff, but they could clearly see that it hadn't been inserted properly to begin with. I had suffered enough, and when they saw the condition that my arm was now in, they could then clearly see what the issue had been.

Each morning in the ward the nurse would approach each patient's bed to have a needle injection inserted into their stomach. I could clearly see that some patients had developed severe yellow and purple bruising from receiving this injection every day. I enquired from the nursing staff as to what was the reason, why this injection was being given to patients? I was told that it was to stop DVT or Deep Vein Thrombosis, which was known to develop as a result of lying in bed all day long.

I said under no circumstances did I want that injection given to me, as I would not be lying in bed all day long. Every morning after that, and before breakfast, I would get up, put on my dressing gown and my blue suede slippers and push the IV drip trolley, with the wheels attached, outside into the nearby courtyard. There I would exercise for around thirty minutes, walking around and around the courtyard like a young pony being broken in. It reminded me of my dad breaking in horses in nearby fields when I was a child.

After a while I got to know the cleaning staff personally and it was nice to spend some time chatting with them each morning in the small canteen attached to my ward and having the morning news on the Television in the background.

The hospital breakfast was really bad, and on several occasions, I managed to elope down the rear hospital fire stairwell, in my dressing gown and blue suede slippers and I walked outside of the building to a nearby Hungry Jack's store to get some breakfast, that wasn't only just a slice of white bread and jam.

On two separate occasions at the hospital, I had managed to contract two different viruses. The first one was the Norovirus, which is usually only contracted on cruise ships. I was told. "You must have picked it up at home somewhere." I said, "I haven't seen anybody since I was last here, and I don't go on cruise ship holidays for that reason, that I don't want to get sick from encountering other people's germs.

On another hospital stay I managed to contract the Rotavirus. Once again, I knew that this was a virus that was usually only contractible, from younger children. As I hadn't been near any young children, I knew that I had contracted this virus during my stay in the hospital. At this stage I was now becoming more fearful of attending the hospital. One of the benefits however, of having a virus in the hospital is that you get to stay in your own private room.

This is because you are apparently 'contagious' to everyone else around you, including nurses, caterers and the cleaners that enter your room. You are a patient that everyone tries to avoid having any contact with.

They are all dressed as if a sudden nuclear attack is imminent, as they all enter the room wearing face masks, gowns, eye wear, special shoes and surgical gloves. One funny incident that occurred in the ward, just before I contracted any of the viruses, was in the early hours one morning.

Just when I thought everyone else was asleep in their beds I left my own bed, which at this time was surrounded by the constant beep, beep, beep, of everyone else's intravenous drip machines going haywire in the ward, to go to the nearby ward toilet. I had my eye mask pushed up onto my forehead as I used it at night-time to help me to get to sleep.

This was due to the lights in the ward only being very slightly dimmed and they remained very visible, making it quite difficult to sleep at night. As I reopened the toilet door into the dimly lit ward there was an elderly patient standing outside at the door. It was around 2.00am. He suddenly panicked at the sight of the mask on my forehead, and he then said to me "I thought you were Zorro."

This was a reference to a figure from a television programme many years ago which was called 'The Mask of Zorro.' It was a funny incident, and we both laughed before going back to our own beds again.

I was really struggling now with my health. My weight had dropped dramatically from a normal level of eighty-two kilos, down to only a mere fifty-two kilos. I was starting to develop cachexia, from losing so much weight rapidly each day. I couldn't stop the shocking weight loss which was being caused by the constant non-stop diarrhoea that I was experiencing. It was terrible. I told the oncologist that I suspected that the combination treatment had triggered an auto-immune condition known as colitis, which was an inflammation within my colon.

I was told that this was rubbish and that's not possible, and it's just something that you must have eaten. I knew this wasn't the case as I had all the symptoms, which I had previously researched in advance and the initial reason that I was trying to avoid having this therapy in the very first place.

I requested a hospital colonoscopy to prove my point. This was subsequently refused, so at this stage I told the specialist that I would discharge myself from the hospital immediately and I would have a private colonoscopy carried out, to prove that I was indeed suffering from a chronic form of colitis, that I believed, had been triggered from receiving both the Opdivo and the Yervoy infusions.

At this point there was a sudden change of mind, quite possibly from the imminent embarrassment, that could have been caused, from the results of an outsourced procedure.

It was agreed that I would be allowed to have a colonoscopy within the hospital itself. The next morning, I was taken to the hospital Gastroenterology department. Shortly after I arrived, I undressed from my hospital pyjamas once again and got dressed into the theatre gown, which I would be required to wear for the procedure. At this stage I spoke to the specialist who was going to perform the procedure, regarding what I believed was going on with my colon and I asked him "Please can you use as much care as you possibly can, as I am completely raw at this stage."

Within a few hours of the biopsy procedure being carried out, the results came back to the hospital ward confirming that yes, I had indeed tested positive for mild colitis. My instincts had once again proven to be correct. The oncologist then decided at this stage to increase the usual prescriptions of Imodium and Gastro-stop.

These once again were all the medications that I had already been taking for almost six weeks and with which I had not achieved any success. I requested to be discharged home as I felt I was probably going to die within the hospital, if I remained there much longer.

My friends who had come to visit me could all clearly see what was developing, from the state that I was now in. I had already tried what is known as the BRAT recommendation of Banana, Rice, Applesauce and Toast. Once again, I not been able to achieve any success from this protocol. I decided at this point that I would discharge myself from the hospital and just go home. I was still in a very bad way at this point, but I was still alive, albeit barely.

I contacted the people in Latvia with whom I had been corresponding with, regarding the Rigvir treatment and the lady I spoke with there, told me about a product that she had previously used for her own children at school when they developed severe diarrhoea. I started to research the product, which I found was a Basonite clay powder called Smecta. It was used to help dry up an inflamed colon. I tried to order it within Australia but unfortunately it wasn't available anywhere.

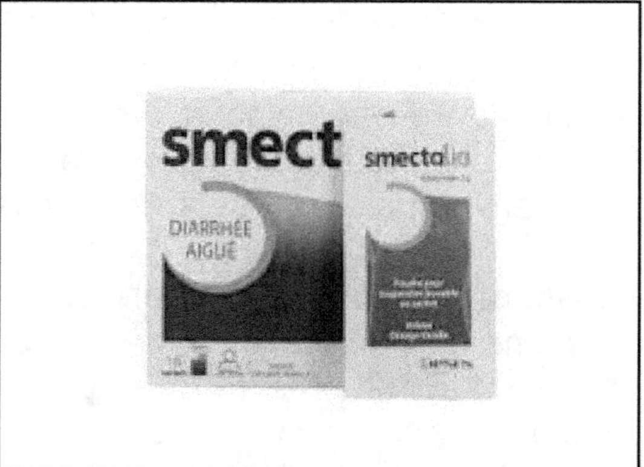

**The Smecta Powder that I found which stopped
over 6 weeks and 30 kilos of weight loss**

A friend Chris, who just happened to be in Thailand at that time, as his wife was attending a conference there. I contacted Chris to see if he could purchase it for me in the local chemists there, who I knew stocked it, and if he could bring it back with him to Australia. I can look back now and laugh at this moment, even though I had a near death experience happening at the very same time. Chris asked me "What am I bringing back for you Rob?" I said, "It's ok, mate trust me, it's nothing illicit, or illegal." We both laughed together at this funny conversation that we both just had. Chris returned to Australia a few days later and drove straight from the airport to my house with the medication.

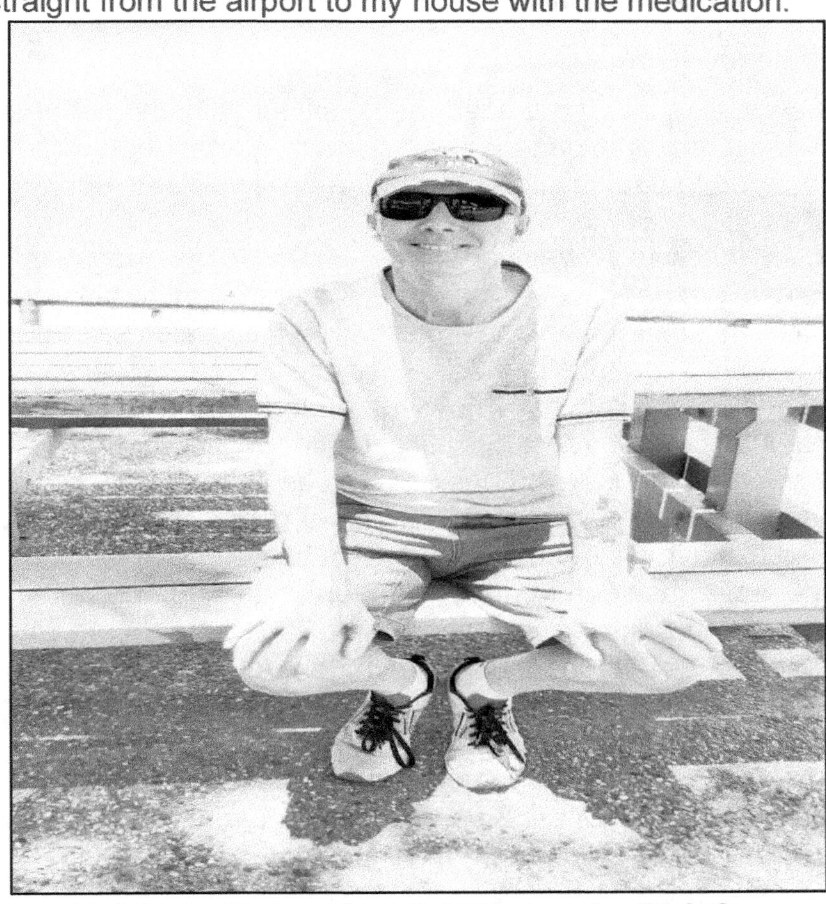

Robin in November 2017 at only 52 kilos

I was so ill at this time that I couldn't even manage to get out of my bed. My wife collected the treatment from Chris at the door of the house and brought it straight to me in bed. I started taking it straight away and within only a few days I was able to get up out of bed and walk around the house once again.

I was amazed, as I had spent the last six weeks in the hospital and nothing there had helped me to control this whatsoever, only the fact that I had been able to prove to them my own diagnosis of colitis. I contacted the lady in Latvia to thank her very much for her help in saving my life once again.

A few weeks later I attended the hospital again and I shared my most recent experience with them, regarding how I had managed to heal my colitis using the Smecta treatment.

Again, this was viewed very dimly, but I was very happy to share my experience, in the hope, that it might just help others, at some point in the future, who might also be in a similar situation to what I was in. I have since discovered that many hospitals have now started to prescribe it to their patients and that a recent clinical trial of the treatment has proven that it is indeed considered to be a cure for colitis in many different countries! To me, it had certainly been a very good discovery indeed. My treatment had been halted at this time, as it was seen to be too dangerous to continue with it, as it was now attacking my body, in a similar fashion to what had previously happened in December 2014, when I had suffered the SIRS attack, at the same hospital.

Some people had managed to achieve success with this treatment, however most patients had not, and in fact quite a few patients had died from receiving it.

Later, on the 20th of November 2019, after their own reviews, the drug manufacturer BMS admitted, that their drugs had failed in a large percentage of patients, compared with just prescribing Opdivo (Nivolumab) by itself alone, as a single agent drug and not used as a combination treatment with the Yervoy (Ipillumab).

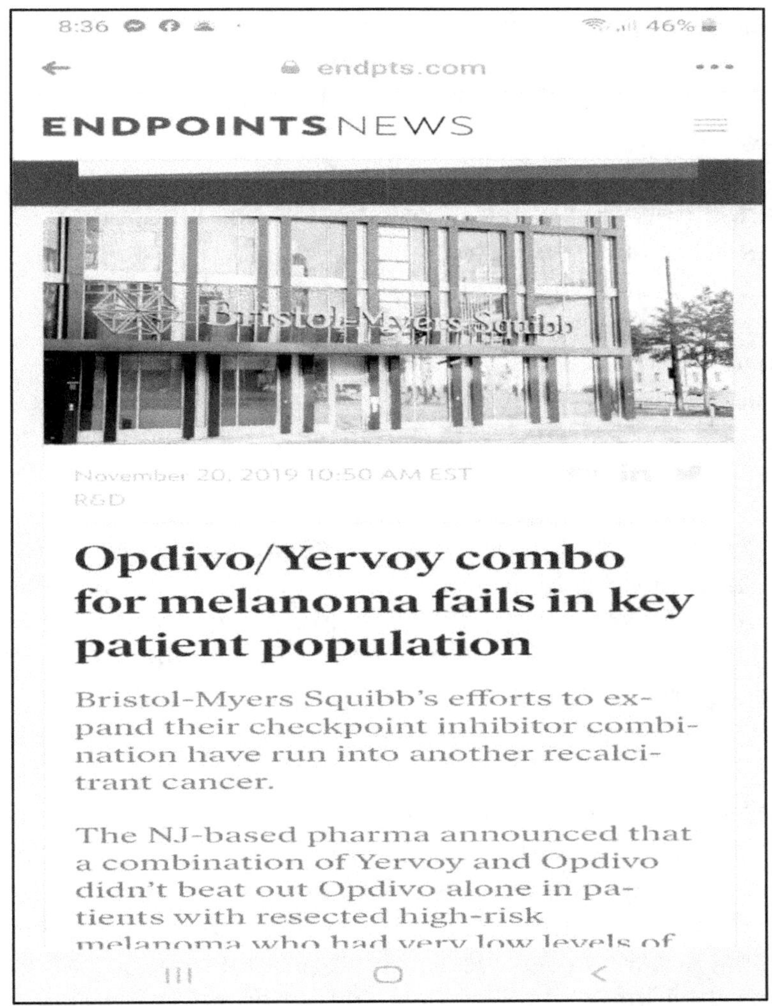

ENDPOINTS NEWS

November 20, 2019 10:50 AM EST
R&D

Opdivo/Yervoy combo for melanoma fails in key patient population

Bristol-Myers Squibb's efforts to expand their checkpoint inhibitor combination have run into another recalcitrant cancer.

The NJ-based pharma announced that a combination of Yervoy and Opdivo didn't beat out Opdivo alone in patients with resected high-risk melanoma who had very low levels of

The company's own admission that their Opdivo alone had beaten their Yervoy combination

I needed to start looking now at ways to rebuild my body again, as it had been virtually destroyed by this latest treatment, which I had been the most fearful off from the very beginning.

From my throat, down to my stomach and then to my colon, had been destroyed, and the weight loss that I had developed, dropping from eighty-two kilos down to only fifty-two kilos, had been massive. I had lost over thirty kilos in only six weeks, and I no longer had any clothing left that would fit me.

I started travelling to the Gold Coast at this time, where I began attending a private clinic at Robina. The doctor there prescribed me a mixed blend of Amino Acids (less the Glutamine, which I knew promoted cancer) and I also received various infusions, to try to help me repair and rebuild, as I was now extremely weak. I carried out more research and I started to take a protein supplement called Fortisip.

This was a product that I already knew was available in Australia, and contained very little sugar content and which was also packed with all the vitamins and minerals that my body desperately needed right now, to help it rebuild itself once again.

I had previously been given other products at the hospital which were packed with sugars, which I already knew fed the cancer cells and none of them had been shown to help me in any way. I remembered back to the period when I was first given the chemotherapy. During this toxic period, the hospital snacks trolley would come around to each patient during their infusions. They would be offered soft drinks, lollies, and chocolate.

In fact, everything that was packed full of sugar that was indeed, just feeding the cancer in their bodies, that they were trying to eradicate.

At one stage I even sent a letter addressed directly to the hospital dietician, requesting that healthy alternatives be offered to cancer patients from the snacks trolley. Instead of being offered sugar products, which were making people's cancers progress worse.

The Fortisip compact protein supplement that I selected for myself in November 2017, I still take each day, and it's one that I have also recommended to many other people, to help them rebuild successfully from similar situations.

I had additional private blood tests completed, which I then sent to the RGCC testing centre in Greece, at another cost of ten thousand dollars. I was certainly trying everything at this point.

The idea behind this test was that RGCC might just be able to produce a vaccine that could help me continue to fight my cancer.

I had a vaccine produced by the laboratory in Greece, which was then delivered to the cancer clinic on the Gold Coast. I travelled to the clinic over several weeks to have it administered in the hope that it might bring me some success, but sadly once again, this wasn't to be.

I was now quickly running out of options again, and with no further medical treatments being made available to me, I didn't know what I could do next. I started my own investigations and research, searching for alternative methods, to try to help me continue to survive on this personal cancer journey.

I researched Vitamin C infusions, which I had administered each week over several months at the Gold Coast clinic. I ordered more of the mistletoe extract (Helixor) treatment from Germany and once again I had this administered intravenously each week.

I ordered more of the Rigvir Echo-7 viral preparation from Latvia, but as I already knew it wasn't an FDA approved treatment, then it would probably be denied entry into Australia at the various customs border points.

I decided to apply for a concession from the relevant government department in Canberra, to allow me to try it, as I had no other medical options left available to me at this time. My own GP assisted me with completing the application for an import permit, but it was again refused even though it was for my own personal use. In fact, I rang the relevant department in Canberra, who issued the permits directly, and I pleaded with them, that I may be allowed to bring this treatment to Australia, to help me try to save my own life, as there was absolutely nothing else left for me to try at this point.

In their first denial, they told me that it was being refused because there were already melanoma treatments available in Australia. I replied by telling them that I was already aware of this, but I was being refused the treatment, by all the oncologists at the public hospitals.

The lady's response was simply to tell me that maybe now might be the right time to start to get all my affairs into order, and did I have a valid Will in place? I was astounded at this, and I felt so humiliated. I was even more surprised the very next day, when she rang me back again to apologise for the way that she had spoken to me the day before. It was obvious, that her demeanour had affected her sleep pattern that very same night.

I decided at this time not to give up, so I started a Petition, and all my friends signed it. The permit was finally approved, and I was granted permission to import the trial treatment.

As the viral preparation had to be transported in dry ice via a special medical courier, to keep the vaccine at the required temperature of minus twenty degrees for its survival, and to prevent it from being spoilt, the courier cost was extremely expensive.

The medical courier unfortunately could only arrange to transport the treatment from Riga in Latvia to Sydney, which then became a fourteen-hour drive from my home, and then another fourteen hours return trip back home again. I managed to get a friend to collect it for me in Sydney, and they placed it into their own portable medical fridge. They left Sydney with my treatment, and we arranged to meet each other at Coffs Harbour on the North Coast of New South Wales, at a well-known tourist spot called The Big Banana.

Here we swapped over the treatment, which at this stage was still packed in the original dry ice, that it had been transported in from Latvia and I used my own portable medical fridge to transport it back home in my own vehicle.

After the fourteen-hour drive back to Queensland again, I removed the fridge from my vehicle and I plugged it straight into the mains supply and attached the emergency device that I had already prepared in the event of a power failure.

MORE MEDICAL BLUNDERS AHEAD

I decided I would continue to try having Acupuncture treatment again, and I had this therapy carried out once a week for several months. In December 2017, after another whole-body scan at the hospital in Brisbane, a swollen tissue was seen in the medical imaging scan on my salivary gland, which was just in front of my left ear. I discussed this with the oncologist and we both agreed that in order to prove that it really was another cancer tumour a needle biopsy might be a better way forward, instead of just guessing from the recent scanned images. The biopsy was arranged at the hospital for 16th Jan 2018, and this would be carried out under a fine needle guided aspirate, to define if it was indeed a cancerous tumour, or if it was just only a normal piece of body fatty tissue.

At the same time, I decided to make another appointment to attend the Peter Mac Cancer centre in Melbourne for some further second opinions regarding my current situation, with having no treatment being offered to me by any oncologist.

I flew to Melbourne on the 5th of January 2018 to attend this meeting. When I returned to Brisbane, the date had already been arranged for me to have my salivary gland biopsy carried out on the 16th of January 2018, under an ultrasound guided procedure within the hospital Pathology department in Brisbane. In fact, not just one, but three individual needles were injected through the side of my face into the salivary gland, to draw out the necessary cells required for testing.

Each needle was pierced through my cheek into my salivary gland, and the specimen cells that had been extracted, were then placed onto a glass slide, which was then sent to the hospital pathology laboratory to have further tests carried out and a full analysis report prepared.

Here the extracted cells would then undergo further analysis, which would enable them to test it, and to produce a report detailing their findings. The result came back later as being highly suspicious of a Metastatic Melanoma tumour. I was then referred to the hospital surgeon to discuss the removal of the salivary gland. After a discussion with this hospital surgeon, I felt very uncomfortable with what his approach was going to be, regarding the surgical removal of my gland.

I sought an appointment immediately with my own GP, to express my concerns regarding how this planned surgery was going to be carried out. My GP suggested that I should discuss this further with my Ear, Nose and Throat surgeon and specialist, who I attended on the Sunshine Coast. I followed his advice, and I contacted my Ear, Nose and Throat specialist for an appointment. He informed me that, he could indeed perform the procedure at the Buderim Private hospital the following week. The registrar then provided me with an estimated cost of the surgery, the hospital, the theatre room and the anaesthetist costs.

The total amount was ten thousand dollars. He also informed me that he would obtain the previously scanned images, as well as a copy of the hospital pathology report, and then, out of medical courtesy, he would call the hospital surgeon in Brisbane to personally discuss with him what his intended plans were going to be for the removal of my salivary gland.

After this, he would then contact me again, to discuss the result of his chat.

He called me back a few days later, to inform me that since our last conversation he had indeed spoken with the surgeon in Brisbane, and he then continued to explain what had been discussed between them both.

He told me that in his own opinion the planned hospital surgery would leave me looking like a stroke victim. That side of my face where the salivary gland was located, would have a deep hole cut into it, like a golf bunker and because of the nerve detail in that part of my face, he didn't know how it would be possible to re-join all the nerves again, using the method that the surgeon had described to him over the phone.

The result could be, that my left eye and the left side of my mouth would be permanently drooped, and that I probably wouldn't be able to blink from my left eye again properly. I would most likely always have different facial expressions as well.

This was astounding and I was very relieved that once again I had sought a second opinion at this time. I asked him if he carried out the operation what would be his procedure to remove my salivary gland. He informed me that his approach would be to cut a line from the front of my ear, and he would then continue this cut around the back of my ear and down the left side of my neck. This would allow him to peel my face back and then remove my salivary gland which was located underneath it. This way he could work carefully with the nerves to ensure that they weren't damaged, and by so doing, it would avoid any long term and permanent damage being caused to that side of my face.

I felt slightly more comfortable with this approach, and I agreed that this seemed to be a more appropriate way to remove it, rather than just simply cutting a large hole into my face through my cheek. I then asked him if it would be possible to receive a sample of the removed tumour once the surgery had been completed, as I would like to send it to a laboratory in Germany known as Therapy Select, to undergo genetic testing. The reason behind sending the tumour to Germany was that during my treatment in Berlin, the doctor whom I attended with, told me that this was the laboratory where all his tissue samples were being sent for testing and he highly recommended their work.

He said this would be the best laboratory to use, in order to see which treatments might be more suitable for the patient to respond with. After my terrible experiences previously, I thought that this was a more personalised, practical and sensible approach, rather than just trying to use a one size fits all approach.

I believed then, that this was something that all hospitals should consider implementing going forward, as not everyone responds in a similar manner. We are all different through nature.

The following week I was admitted to the Buderim Private hospital on the Sunshine Coast for yet another surgical procedure. I was taken to the operating theatre, and I awoke several hours later surrounded by drip tubes, oxygen hoses in my nose and a drainage tube coming out of my neck.

I was back in the ward once again, and I was very relieved that it was all over. The next morning the surgeon came around to see me in my hospital bed and he informed me that the operation had been successful and that the salivary gland tissue had been removed and he had taken it personally to the Pathology laboratory within the hospital.

Here at the laboratory the removed salivary gland would then be tested once again, to confirm that it was indeed cancerous, as the previous three needle aspirates from the pathology report in Brisbane said it was suspicious of another metastatic melanoma.

He suggested that in order to save me the extra expense of spending yet another night in the hospital, that I should be discharged, and the drainage tube would be placed into a bag, which I could then attach to my belt, and which he would remove from my neck the next day in his own practice. I agreed to this, and I left the ward with the blood-filled bag attached to my trouser belt. He said, "I will also have your tumour specimen prepared for you tomorrow, and it will be embedded in paraffin wax to preserve it." "The laboratory will retain a portion for their own records, and the remainder of the tumour, you can then send to the laboratory in Germany for your genetic testing." I thanked him for his help.

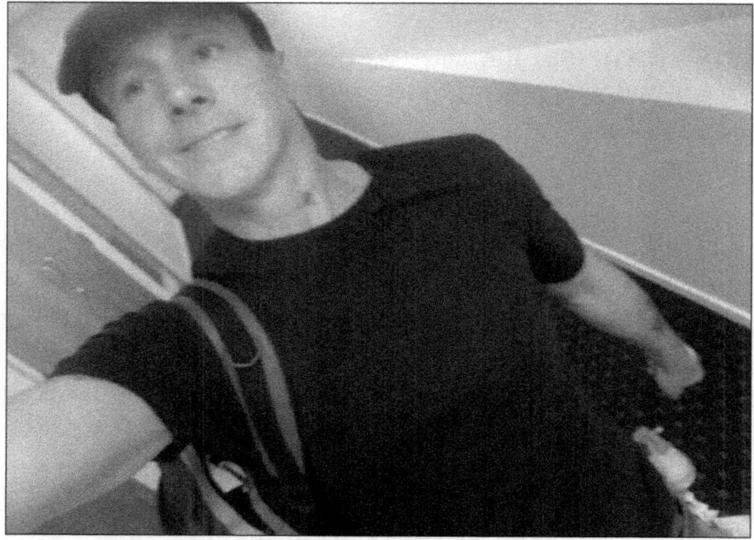

Robin leaving the hospital with the neck tube pushed into a plastic bag

The next day I returned to the clinic, but as I was early for my appointment, I decided to go for a coffee in the nearby Kawana shopping centre. I still had the drainage tube dangling from my neck at this stage, so I put the blood-filled drainage container into a plastic shopping bag, and I carried it through the shopping centre, to conceal it from public view. I saw the surgeon in his practice, and he pulled the tube out from the site of the salivary gland removal in my face, down through my neck.

He then stitched that part of my neck, where the tube had exited through. I left the tube, drainage bag and shopping bag in his practice for disposal.

I had already prepaid six thousand dollars to the laboratory in Germany as an upfront payment for the testing and analysis of the removed salivary gland, which I was now arranging to send.

I was having trouble trying to find a suitable courier who was prepared to transport a 'body part,' as there were very few couriers who would accept a human body part. Two days later I received a telephone call from the Ear Nose and Throat surgeon who had performed the operation. He asked me "Are you sitting down?" I replied, "No, why do you ask me that?" He then asked me if I had sent the tumour specimen over to Germany yet for the testing. I said "No, I haven't as yet as I am actually having difficulty trying to find a courier company who will accept carrying a body part." He then shocked me completely. He said "I understand the initial needle biopsy was taken three times. Is that correct?"

I replied "Yes, that's correct three fine needle aspirates were taken from the salivary gland for pathological analysis at the hospital in Brisbane, as per the report that you received."

He said, "Well don't bother sending it to Germany, it wasn't a malignant tumour after all, it was only just a cyst." I was in total shock. I said, "How on earth could that happen?" I could maybe understand one or even two needle aspirates being wrong, but three was totally beyond belief. He said that in all his thirty years of being a surgeon and carrying out multiple operations he had never known a pathology report to be so wrong. I was devastated again. My whole face had been disfigured, I no longer had any saliva in that side of my mouth, as the salivary gland was now gone, but I had been very lucky indeed, as the outcome, could have been a lot worse for me should the operation have been carried out at the hospital in Brisbane using their surgeon, as was the original plan. Again, if you are ever in any doubt then you should always seek a second opinion.

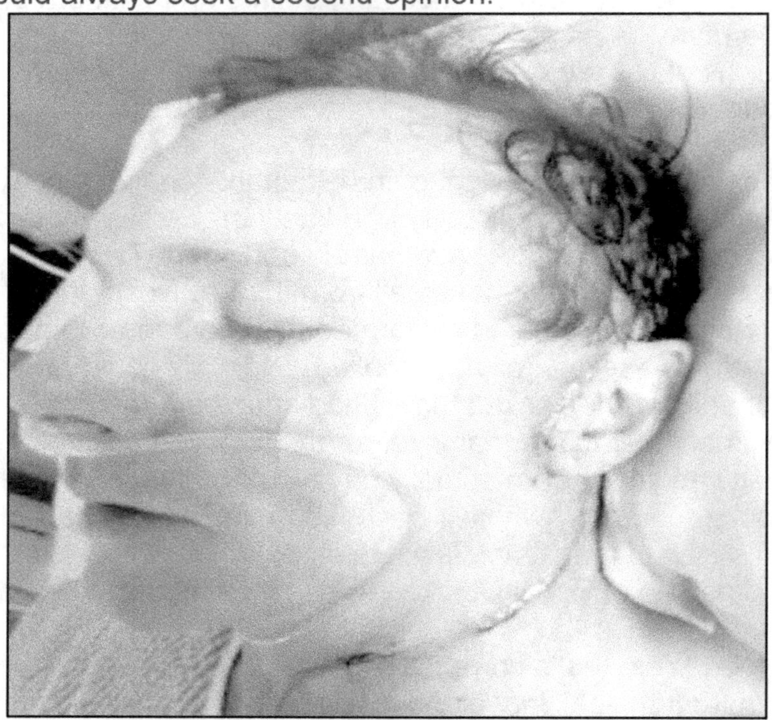

After 3 Needle Tests and Biopsies said you have Salivary Gland Cancer, it was only a cyst.

Immediately, I contacted the Therapy Select laboratory in Germany, to explain to the professor, that the so called 'cancer tumour' that I was trying to send him for testing, was in fact not a cancer tumour after all, but it was only just a 'cyst,' and that the sample would not be sent to them for testing, as it would be pointless, analysing a normal piece of tissue which was not even cancerous. He agreed and understood this, however, I was unable to receive a refund on the six thousand dollars that I had already prepaid, and it was recorded as a future credit on my existing medical file at the laboratory. I returned to the hospital in Brisbane two weeks later, to try to find out how a pathology report could be so wrong.

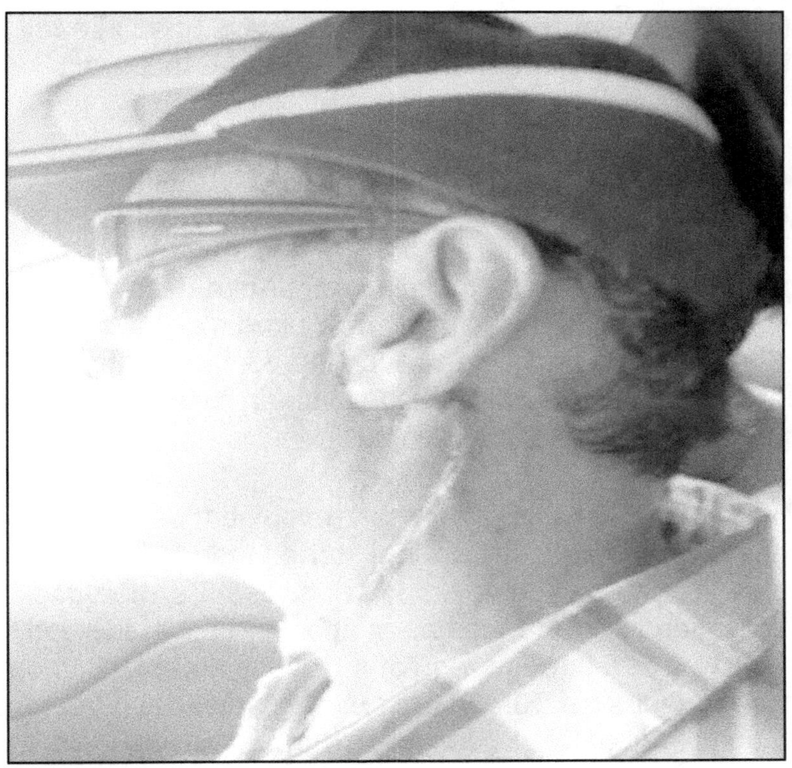

Going back to the hospital, to ask how they got a Biopsy so wrong after 3 Needle Tests

Three needle aspirates had been taken, and all the unnecessary pain, torment, trauma, disfigurement and expense that I had endured once again, had all been in vain.

Unfortunately, there were no answers forthcoming, and I did not receive any explanation as to how this could possibly have happened to me.

I decided that with no other hospital treatment options available to me now, just to continue with my mistletoe extract infusions (Helixor) and my Rigvir vaccine injections.

I continued to have these carried out each week for the next few months, again at a cost of approximately ten thousand dollars, which was in addition to the outlays I had already paid earlier for the treatment of one hundred thousand dollars.

In April 2018 I had another whole-body PET scan carried out at the same Brisbane hospital. With no treatment options being given or even offered to me at this stage, the scan had apparently shown that a muscle tumour had developed on the side of my thigh, which was now almost eight centimetres long and it was becoming very uncomfortable to sleep with and especially difficult to sit anywhere, as it now resembled the size of a tennis ball.

In September 2018, another scan revealed that I now had three new tumours in my brain. I started researching again for several hours each day, and I had read up where the thymus gland in cattle, had been shown to boost the body's immune system through regular injections. I decided to order this treatment from Europe, and once it arrived, I began the injections at home each day into my arm. I have always had a phobia of needles, so injecting myself each day wasn't an easy thing to do.

The scan had also shown that I had a new tumour now in my lower chest which measured fifteen millimetres in length.

I decided at this time, if I was to have this removed, I could try once again to send it to the laboratory in Germany to have it tested, for any possible future treatment options as there was nothing being offered to me now at the hospital.

It would also give me an opportunity to use up my six-thousand-dollar credit from the laboratory, which was remaining after the previous salivary gland negligence.

I was told by the oncologist that maybe now was the right time to consider going instead to Palliative Care, as I was running out of any further treatment options, as the disease was progressing very rapidly and very soon, I would be suffering a lot more pain.

I refused this option as I felt that by doing this I was giving in totally to the disease, and I refused to go to Palliative Care, at least for now anyway.

At this point I requested if the small tumour showing up on my lower right chest could be removed for genetic testing. The oncologist replied "Well, this didn't work for you the last time you did this, did it? I said, "What do you mean by this?" "Well, you got a dodgy Sunshine Coast back yarder to remove it for you, who then stuck it into a jam jar." I was shocked that a specialist would say this about another specialist with over forty years of surgical experience. I replied by saying that I was very dismayed that you would refer to a well-respected surgeon in this way and it was your original pathology testing in the very first place that had confirmed, after three needle aspirates had been taken, that it was a suspicious Metastatic Melanoma tumour, and it turned out to have only just been a fatty cyst. I said, "the blunder started with you."

I also said, "that if I had of allowed the hospital surgeon to carry out the removal, as you had planned, not only would I have no salivary gland but my face, would have been terribly disfigured." The entire procedure had been totally pointless and both very expensive and disfiguring for me.

In October 2018, I attended the Brisbane hospital once more for a day surgery procedure to remove the small fifteen-millimetre tumour from my right lower chest.

I was taken to the hospital ward, where I was prepared for the operation in the usual fashion, by changing into the theatre gown and having the blue net cap fitted onto my head. This was to be a day only procedure, carried out under a local anaesthetic.

So instead of being fully anaesthetised and put out to sleep, I was only injected into the lower chest area, where the surgery was going to be carried out. Afterwards, I was so glad and extremely thankful that this had indeed been the case.

I was placed onto a theatre bed, and the area that was to be excised for the tumour removal was brush smeared with the usual purple iodine, which was to try to reduce the risk of any infections occurring after the operation. I received several local anaesthetic injections into my lower right chest, which was then cut open and the tumour was removed. I asked the surgeon at this point, if I could please see the tumour that he had just removed from my chest. He showed me the tumour, and I was shocked at what had just been taken from my lower chest.

The tissue portion that he had just removed resembled the size of an egg.

I asked the surgeon, as to what was the reason why, such a large amount of tissue had just been removed, considering that the size of the tumour was only fifteen millimetres. This piece that had been cut out was approximately five centimetres or two inches in diameter.

He replied that it was a necessary procedure, to ensure that all the cancer had been removed to provide 'clear margins.'

I looked curiously at the black and grey coloured tumour in the centre of the removed tissue, as I had never actually seen a tumour outside of the body before.

Nevertheless, I was still concerned that such a huge section of body tissue had been removed from my chest, just to extract a small fifteen-millimetre tumour. After this, the surgeon said to me, "Okay, now roll over onto your right side, so I can remove the muscle tumour from the top of your thigh and hip as well."

I said "No, you won't." He then replied, "It's in your theatre surgery paperwork, that both your lower chest tumour and your thigh muscle tumour are both to be removed today."

I told the surgeon "If you need to remove that amount of tissue from my chest cavity, which is almost the size of an egg, just to extract a fifteen-millimetre tumour, how much are you going to remove from my leg, to extract a tumour which is the size of a tennis ball?" His reply again astounded me. He said, "Well you won't be able to walk again normal, you will probably require the use of a walking stick, to help you to retain your balance." I said, "Isn't this something that you should have discussed with me before the surgery, and not something that I would have only found out later, if I actually had been fully anaesthetised and when I would awaken, only to discover that it was then too late?"

He didn't reply to this question. I got up from where I was lying on the theatre bed, and I removed the blue net cap I was wearing on my head, and I placed it back down on the bed. I looked over towards the surgeon standing in his blue theatre gown, cap and mask, holding his scalpel, and I said to him, "I'm leaving here right now. You have taken enough out of me today. I will see you later." I walked out of the theatre still dressed in the gown that I had walked in wearing and I got myself dressed back into my normal clothing once again and I left the hospital to make my way back home. As I drove home, I was very thankful that I had not been fully anaesthetised for this procedure, otherwise I would never have been able to walk out of the hospital or even drive a vehicle again.

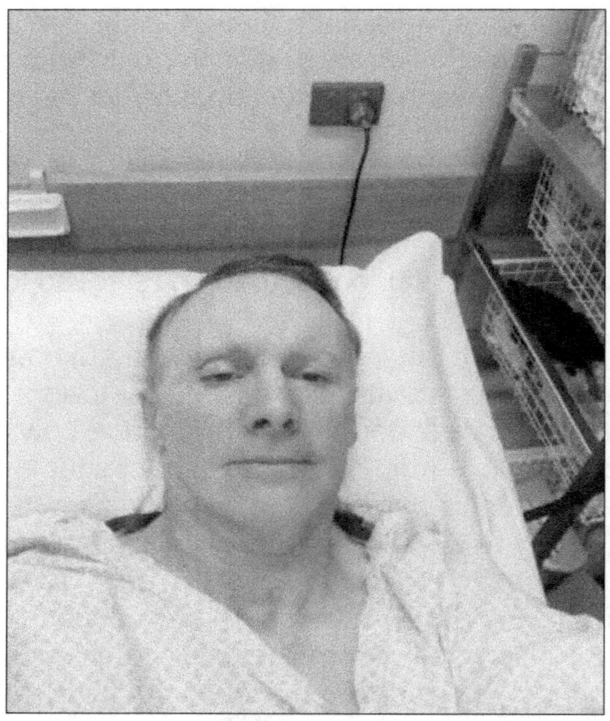

Awaiting the Chest Tumour removal for testing

FIGHT YOUR OWN CORNER

Several days later I contacted the hospital, to request a sample of my tumour from the pathology department. I had already explained to them, before agreeing to have the procedure carried out, that I wanted to send it overseas to a laboratory in Germany, known as Therapy Select. This is where the tumour would be genetically tested, to try to find out which treatment I might just respond to, in a continued effort to extend my life. I was told that it was now the property of the hospital, and that they couldn't release it back to me. I told them that you can retain a portion of it in your laboratory, which I fully understand is your standard procedure after any operation has been completed, however it's also actually a part of my own physical body, which you have removed, and it really does belong to me. Again, my request was denied. The next day I drove back to Brisbane and went to the hospital.

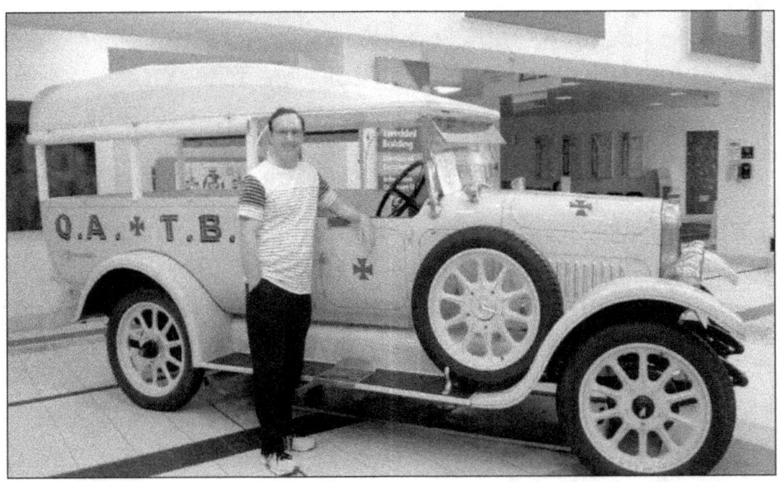

Back at the hospital looking for my own tumour to send to Germany for Genetic testing

103

Upon entering the entrance foyer, I walked over to the main information desk, where I requested from the attendant as to how I might be able to find my way to the pathology department of the hospital. After receiving this information from the lady at the desk, I avoided using the lifts, due to the risk of picking up germs as the lifts were always packed with people and I then proceeded to climb up the stairwell. After I reached the pathology floor level, I continued to walk along several corridors until I finally reached the pathology department.

At the pathology reception desk, I explained to the receptionist who I was and why I was there, as it wasn't a department of the hospital that was normally frequented by non-nursing staff. Again, I was told sorry, but we can't release it to you as it's now officially the property of the hospital from here on. I said it belongs to me, and you have just removed it from my body for pathological testing and I would like it returned now please, as I want it tested again overseas, in an attempt, to save my own life. I explained that this was the reason I had given my consent for its removal in the very first place. At this point, I requested to speak to the head of the hospital Pathology department, however once again this request was denied. I told the receptionist, "I will be back again tomorrow with the exact same request. I won't go away you know."

I returned to the hospital the next day and I went through the exact same ritual as I had experienced the previous day. I informed the Pathology department that I was being denied the opportunity to try to save my own life and that this was so wrong and probably highly illegal as well.

I told them that my next point of contact would be with the director of the hospital, as I wasn't wasting any more time trying to deal with the Pathology department.

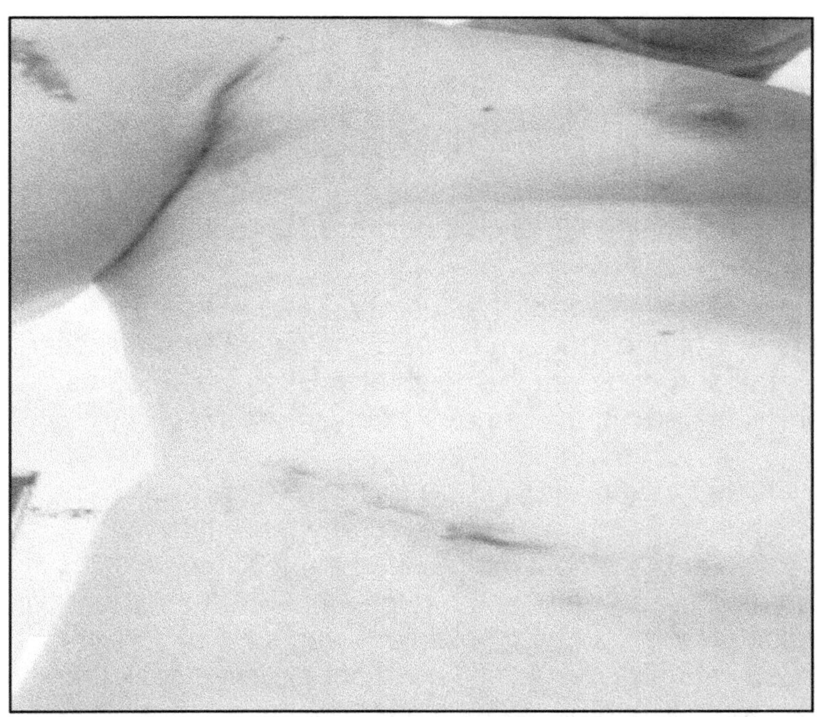

The huge scar left removing the 10mm Tumour

I returned home again, and I immediately started to write a personal letter addressed to the director of the hospital, explaining my situation, and that if the tumour wasn't returned to me, then I would report the matter to one of the local news stations, who would be very pleased to highlight my plight, by taking it to air in Queensland. Two days later I received a reply from the director of the hospital, requesting the address details of the laboratory in Germany, where the tumour was to be sent to, and informing me that they would courier it there directly, on my behalf from the hospital. Finally, some common sense had prevailed, and with this latest news I informed the professor at Laboratory Select in Germany, that the tumour biopsy would very soon be on its way to Germany to have the genetic testing carried out. that I had already paid for, and I looked forward to receiving the test results from them as soon as possible.

I contacted the hospital again a few days later to follow up on the matter, and they confirmed that the tumour tissue was now in the mailing section of the hospital awaiting collection, and that I would be sent the courier tracking information by email, once it became available to them.

A few weeks later after the surgery, I was at home one day when my phone rang. I answered the call only to discover it was the surgeon from the hospital in Brisbane who had earlier carried out the removal of my chest tumour.

He wanted to know how I was going after the procedure, and he then asked me if I needed any more tumours removed at this time. I appreciated the follow up call regarding the surgery, as I had previously left the theatre on strained terms with him, however I was quite simply amazed that any surgeon would call a patient directly to ask them if they would like to have any more tumours removed.

To me, it seemed most unusual that a surgeon would ring a patient directly looking to carry out further work on them. I would have expected that a specialist would liaise with a surgeon first, on behalf of a patient, who may be requiring some form of surgical procedure to be carried out, but not a surgeon calling the patient personally and asking this question. I said, "Thank you for your offer, however I'm okay at this stage." He then told me. "Well, you know where to find me if you need me."

In November the sample tumour finally arrived at Therapy Select in Germany. From here it would be tested with a variety of different treatments, to see which one or ones that my cancer might succeed in responding with. Several treatments tested positive for a favourable response with the tumour, but one was a combination treatment, that I had previously responded to.

It had also stopped working for me in August 2016. This is the same treatment I had researched earlier in the USA, and the one which I had told the oncologist, could possibly work a second time around, only to be told that my research was rubbish, and no, it wouldn't work again a second time. I said that the latest research had clearly shown that it would.

It was the combination treatment of Tafinlar and Mekinist. The same treatment that today in Australia, is now being prescribed to patients a second time around, albeit for a shorter period, as the cancer cells have a memory and they can very quickly remember how to outsmart the therapy, but it is indeed now being prescribed as a second time around treatment, to many cancer patients. This now gives further hope to others. I was very pleased to learn that this was indeed being prescribed a second time around, after my earlier research had been called rubbish.

Whilst waiting on the tumour results, I decided to continue further investigations into other cancer therapies that were being made available overseas.

I started looking in Mexico, and in China. I contacted the Oasis of Hope hospital in Tijuana, Mexico and another treatment centre at Cancun in Mexico. A good friend of mine Ray, lived nearby in San Diego, and he very kindly offered to help me travel from California County, over the border into Mexico to have the treatment carried out, if I needed to do this. Unfortunately, the treatments, accommodation and travel costs were unaffordable to me. I then decided to contact the New Modern hospital in Guangzhou, which is in the Guangdong province of China as they were producing some good cancer results there, according to their most recent reviews.

Unfortunately, once again the cost was totally prohibitive, as the quotation I was given was in the region of five hundred thousand dollars for just the treatment alone.

In November 2018 a Zoom conference was arranged between me and the professor from the Therapy Select laboratory in Germany.

This conference was to personally discuss with me, the results that he had now received from the tumour genetic testing. The tumour at this stage, had been tested in two different laboratories. One was in Heidelberg in Germany, and the other laboratory was in Phoenix Arizona, in the United States.

During our Zoom conference, the professor confirmed with me that the testing which had been carried out, had shown that the previous combination therapy of Tafinlar and Mekinist could work for me again a second time around.

It had also shown that either of the immunotherapy treatments of Opdivo (Nivolumab) or Keytruda (Pembrolizumab), if given as single agent treatments, could also show positive outcomes for treating my cancer.

I was not prepared to use the combination drug Yervoy (Ippillumab) again, as this was the drug that had almost killed me previously. I contacted the various oncologists once again, both at hospitals in Brisbane and also on the Sunshine Coast, to tell them about my latest tumour testing reports, that I had now received from both the laboratories, and I requested from them both if I could be prescribed either of these two treatments once again, in a continued attempt to try to save my own life.

Unfortunately, my request fell upon deaf ears again and I was told that if I wanted any further treatments then I would have to fund them on my own behalf. I was told that because I had failed these treatments previously, then I can't be provided with them again on the Pharmaceutical Benefits Scheme public system (PBS).

I then started to investigate the cost of these treatments, and the quotations that I received, which would allow me to purchase either of these immunotherapy treatments, was five hundred thousand dollars, and the targeted therapy was thirty-six thousand dollars. I told the oncologists that this was most unfair. I had gone to a huge amount of effort and personal expense to prove to them, that the immunotherapy would indeed work for me once again, but very sadly I was now being denied the opportunity to be treated with them at public hospitals. I told them I already had the operation carried out to remove the initial tumour for testing. Then I had sent it to the laboratory in Germany for testing at a cost of six thousand dollars, and even after all this was completed, I was now still being denied treatment as a patient at a public hospital. It was so wrong.

I said as an Australian citizen, I was now being denied the right to try to save my own life, which was a complete and utter disgrace.

On November 18th I wrote a very personal letter to the Federal health minister in Canberra, pleading to be provided with the Opdivo immunotherapy treatment, that was now readily available in all public hospitals in Australia, as I was still being denied the Keytruda treatment, which was what I really needed. This was being denied to me on the grounds that I had apparently failed on it previously (which I later proved was totally wrong and which left me almost penniless, after being left with no options but to purchase every treatment that I possibly could, in a continued attempt

109

to stay alive) I requested the Opdivo treatment for this reason. I later proved to the oncologists, that this decision to take me off the original Keytruda treatment was completely wrong. The last treatment I had received of Yervoy (Ippilumab), was the only one that I had to cease, as it was the drug which had almost killed me.

I later found out from further research, that it wasn't the actual Opdivo treatment that had caused me the issue, it was the Yervoy treatment, as countless numbers of people had suffered similar side effects to what I had suffered.

I was originally told before commencing this treatment, that after the various cycles of Opdivo (Nivolumab) and Yervoy (Ippilumab) were completed, I would be provided with the Opdivo, as a stand-alone therapy. This never happened and in fact now I was being denied what I had previously been promised. I already knew, that both the Keytruda and the Opdivo were very similar immunotherapy treatments, with the only real difference being, that they were being manufactured by two different pharmaceutical companies.

The recent results from both the laboratories in Germany and in Phoenix, Arizona had now confirmed that my cancer would indeed respond to either of these two treatments, if they were administered to me.

I tried to explain to the oncologists, that it wasn't the Opdivo treatment that had caused me any issues. It had been the Yervoy that had totally devastated me. They said, "No you failed both of them so we can't offer either of them to you again." I had been a working taxpayer for twenty-five years and I felt that public hospital treatment should be made available to me. Sadly, this request was also denied, and the treatment was refused once again, on the later, proved wrongful grounds that I had failed with it before.

Again, searching for help, I discovered treatment that had just become available for Metastatic Melanoma at the Sheba Hospital in Israel, and which was seen to be providing great results for patients trying to overcome this deadly terminal cancer. I contacted the Sheba Hospital, and I received all the latest information regarding the treatments that they offered. It was known as TILS, which stood for Tumour Infiltrating Lymphocytes.

They were able to offer me this treatment but sadly once again the cost was going to be around five hundred thousand dollars which I could not afford to fund myself. I thanked them for sending me their information and I wished them continued success, both with their patients and with their treatments.

I decided to go back to the hospital in Brisbane once again to plead my case and to practically beg for help to try to save my own life.

Again, the treatment which I knew could help me to fight my cancer and which I had proven from the results of the genetic testing at both the laboratories was again refused to me.

Instead, I was told that I should now begin to prepare myself for Palliative Care, which I knew was basically an 'end game' option, to try to reduce my pain, and to assist me to pass on more comfortably.

Instead of providing me with the treatment, which I had already proven would certainly help me, I was instead offered an alternative combination treatment called Vemurafenib and Cobimetinib, which I had previously researched.

I knew that this option would result in horrendous side effects for me, and I wasn't prepared to endure this type of physically torture again. I told the oncologist that this treatment would be too severe on me, and I was told, "Yes you can't go outside when you are on this medication, and if you do decide to go outside then you must wear protective clothing to ensure that every single part of your body is totally covered from head to toe at all times. I suggest that you go to BCF (a large Boating, Camping and Fishing outdoors store) and buy their protective fishing gear and gloves to provide you with all the protection that you will need."

What this now meant was that for me to continue to have any lifestyle left, I would have to be permanently confined indoors, always, and should I decide to leave the house and venture outside, then I was to give the resemblance of the first man landing on the moon. To me neither of these options left me with any form of life, and I rejected them both and left the hospital. I decided to contact some people for a second opinion on the Vemurafenib and Cobimetinib therapy which I had just been offered.

One gentleman told me that his skin had practically all peeled off and he looked like he was suffering from third degree burns.

Another person I contacted, who lived near Noosa on the Sunshine Coast in Queensland, told me that he couldn't even sit near a window, without coming out in a horrendous rash all over his body.

He sent me some pictures of the rash when it happened to him. I had never experienced any side effects like this before with the Tafinlar and Mekinist treatment. The only thing I was told to always avoid with this treatment was eating grapefruit.

Apart from developing SIRS shortly after commencing the treatment I never had any other issues with side effects.

I decided to carry out research on a device called a Frequency Generator GB4000. This was a portable device which was installed in the bedroom of the home. It was positioned beside your bed. It ran all night, emitting various frequency waves towards your body.

This was apparently designed to work in such a way that the cancer cells would be killed by the programmed frequencies, which the generated by the machine.

I decided to order this machine from the USA at a further cost of ten thousand dollars. Sadly, I was to discover later that the online company, with whom I had placed the original order, turned out to be an online fraud scam and I lost my ten thousand dollars. I then started to search again for another machine, and I found a second hand one that was for sale within Australia.

I was able to purchase this machine for seven thousand dollars and I ran the machine daily, using a varied selection of frequency programs that it had been supplied with.

I continued to try this machine for several months, but sadly once again after I had further whole-body scans carried out, the machine had not shown to be helping me in any way, to reduce the spread of my cancer.

I then investigated another frequency machine called a Spooky. This machine had first been introduced to me by a doctor at the Gold Coast clinic. It was a similar device to the previous GB4000 machine however, this machine was connected directly to the body's wrist and ankles, and it could then be set to emit various frequencies directly into my body through the waveforms that it transmitted.

113

I very nervously ordered this machine from overseas at a cost of five thousand dollars, given my concerns regarding the previous online scam, that I had been caught up in already.

The machine arrived okay this time, which was such a relief, however sadly once again, after several months of consistent usage several times each day, I could not seem to accomplish any benefits from using it either.

Still not prepared to give up yet I purchased a pulse zapping machine. This was a device you could carry about with you in your pocket whilst it was connected to your wrist. The idea behind this device was that the various pulses which the machine transmitted could then be pulsed into the veins running through my wrists, as it travelled the entire body's circuit. The idea was to evoke a 'kill' pattern on the cancer cells in the blood stream. The wrist attachment was very uncomfortable to wear, and it always felt that I was receiving constant electric shocks, which were very painful, and I ended up with bad burns on both of my wrists.

I eventually had to stop this procedure, as like the previous ones I did not seem to be benefiting from it, and the result, was simply badly burnt wrists.

Still determined to keep trying to find some other form of help I purchased a body zapper device which resembled a large wand. This worked in a similar manner to a cardiac recovery device.

It was placed on various parts of the body where tumours were located, whilst a large pulse was generated to that part of the body. Again, this was designed to try to get the body to evoke a response against the cancer cell attacks.

I purchased a device that made Coloidial Silver. Others had claimed that this product could improve the immune system to fight off bacteria and viruses.

Once again, I had no success with either of these protocols and all I found that the Colloidal Silver did, was to make me constantly appear looking a greyish colour.

Still trying to find answers, I decided once again to fly to Melbourne in Victoria, to speak with the professor and the oncologists, at the Peter Mac Cancer hospital and to also share with them the results of my most recent tumour testing in Germany.

I explained to them that the only options available to me right now at my local hospitals, were to get my personal affairs in order and go to Palliative Care where I might receive some pain relief, or to try the combination treatment on offer of Vemurafenib and Cobmetinib. The treatment that I really wanted, of either the Keytruda or the Opdivo, were still being denied to me and I had been told, if I wanted either of these two treatments, then I would have to purchase them myself, which I could not afford to do.

I voiced to them my concerns about the side effects of the Vemurafenib and Cobimetinib treatment, and I spoke with them regarding the serious side effects I had suffered previously, and how I had been very close to death with the Yervoy (Ipillumab) treatment.

They all agreed that the Vemurafenib and Cobimetinib treatment might not be the best option for me, unless I lived in the centre of Melbourne. The reason being, that the Victorian weather was usually much harsher and more inclement than the weather in Queensland.

With less daily sunshine and the tall buildings offered more protection from direct sun all day. They told me that in their own personal opinions, it most definitely was not a suitable treatment for me to use residing in Queensland.

Their opinion was rather that, if I could afford to purchase the Tafinlar and Mekinist therapy once again, it might show a more favourable response with less serious side effects. I thanked them once again for their opinions, which I very much appreciated, and I returned to Queensland to further consider my options.

THE SEARCH CONTINUES

I knew at this point that I would not be able to afford the treatment that I really needed, which was the immunotherapy Keytruda or the equivalent immunotherapy treatment Opdivo. I decided to write directly to both pharmaceutical companies regarding the Keytruda and Opdivo treatments, to see if I could be granted compassionate access to either of these two drugs, but very sadly without any success again. They informed me that the request for any treatment had to come directly from an oncologist and not from the patient themselves, which I fully understood and respected.

I then made an appointment with four oncologists at three different hospitals. I asked them if they could access any of these treatments for me, however they informed me that they had already tried to do this and that they didn't have any success. I contacted both the suppliers once again directly, of the Keytruda and the Opdivo and they informed me that they didn't know any of these oncologists and no, they hadn't heard anything from them in relation to trying to obtain compassionate access for me to get their treatments.

This was very upsetting, as up to this point I had already gone through the suffering of having a tumour cut from my chest, which I had sent to Germany for genetic testing, at my own cost of six thousand dollars. I had received the results from this testing which showed that I could respond to either the Keytruda or the Opdivo treatment.

117

I had now shown these results to the various oncologists, and even after doing all this, I was still being refused the treatment that I had been able to prove would help me to fight my cancer.

Up to this point I had also written directly to the Federal Health Minister, I had personally contacted the treatment suppliers, who informed me that this request had to come from the oncologists directly, which I understood and respected. I then approached the oncologists once again to request if they could please write to the suppliers on my behalf to see if the treatments that I have just already proven would help me, could be provided under compassionate access terms. I was then told by these same oncologists that they had already done this on my behalf and now the suppliers were telling me that they didn't know any of these oncologists and neither had they heard from any of them.

This just seemed to be getting worse for me by the day. At this stage I decided to contact the manufacturer of the targeted therapy drugs Tafinlar and Mekinist, to see if they could help me with supplying their treatment on compassionate terms. I also told them that I had been one of their very first patients to trial their combination therapy when it was first launched in 2014. Unfortunately, once again, this request was refused and instead they referred me back to the hospital oncologists again, with a purchase only option.

I had no choice left now, only to try to raise the necessary funding myself, to purchase the Tafinlar and Mekinist targeted treatment directly from the pharmaceutical company. In order to get this treatment process underway, I first had to obtain a hospital prescription from an oncologist.

They needed to authorise the pharmaceutical company to supply the targeted treatment to me and then I had to find a pharmacy who would stock the treatment for me, on a personal basis each month.

I contacted Ramsay Healthcare, who had a pharmacy outlet at a hospital located on the south side of Brisbane. This then became a routine monthly drive, to collect my treatment from this pharmacy. The cost of the combination therapy was almost one thousand dollars per week. For the duration of the treatment being effective again for a second time around, the total cost had amounted to thirty-six thousand dollars.

Some very good friends of mine Chris and Alison kindly assisted me at this time by setting up a Go-Fund me page online and they managed to raise almost ten thousand dollars, which was most appreciated, as my capacity to finance the medication now myself was very minimal, considering the hundreds of thousands of dollars that I had already spent trying to stay alive from using my own savings, my superannuation and then later, finally selling our own family home.

In December 2018 I had another whole-body PET scan at the hospital in Brisbane. The result of this scan showed that there had been a significant increase in the number of tumours throughout my body. This clearly indicated to me, that unless I commenced some other form of therapy very soon, it would be too late for me to try save my life.

I commenced the targeted therapy treatment once again within a few weeks, and I remained on this treatment for another six months, until June 2019.

Sadly, at this time I discovered that the cancer had once again decided to show its ability to outsmart my immune system, and my body had once again stopped responding to it for a second time.

More new tumours had started to appear. I had fully expected that this would be the case from the research that I had carried out earlier into the treatment in the USA.

However, during the six months, I had once again managed to extend my life, as I had been able to reduce the continuous tumour growth. The most recent whole-body scans however confirmed that the combination therapy treatment, sadly was no longer having any effect on my cancer, as it had managed once again to work out how to evade capture and destruction from my body's own immune system soldiers, which were the T cells.

Over the next few months, I tried various other therapies. I continued my daily research, spending hours each day compiling as much information as I possibly could. I tried weekly Vitamin C infusions costing six hundred dollars each treatment, by attending therapy clinics both on the Gold Coast and on the Sunshine Coast. I studied how the thymus gland in cattle had been used to boost the body's own immune system into fighting cancer. I purchased these thymus injections from Europe. Once the treatment arrived, I immediately started to inject these every day into my shoulder muscles. I had also recommenced acupuncture therapy once again every week.

I tried various dietary recommendations including Gerston, Mediterranean, Rainbow, Budwig, plus numerous others. I had already completely cut out all manmade sugars which I already knew, only fed the cancer cells. I lowered my intake of fruit as well, to further reduce even natural sugars.

I had started making green vegetable blended drinks each day, but I had to stop taking them shortly afterwards, as I discovered later that too many raw vegetables can cause fermentation within the body itself.

This results in serious kidney pains, which I began to experience after only a few weeks of commencing these green concoctions. I tried using a solution called DMSO and MSN powder. I mixed them both together into a paste form, which I applied to each tumour. This was very aggressive and hot, and after a few weeks I decided to stop using it as there was no change in the appearance of each tumour.

I purchased another supplement called Gumby Gumby, which was made from the shredded leaves of an Aboriginal tree called Gumby Gumby. I had previously received information, that several people had found this herbal treatment successful in combating their cancers. I used this supplement for several months, but again it did not seem to be helping me in any way to fight my cancer as new tumours kept appearing around my body.

I bought another herbal medicine from the United States called Essiac Tea. It was made from four traditional herbs. These herbs were Burdock Root, Sheep Sorrel, Slippery Elm and Chinese Turkey Rhubarb.

This was an old native Indian tonic. I continue to take this supplement each day, for its cleansing benefits to the body.

I studied how zinger ginger could help to destroy the protective shell which surrounded each cancer cell, leaving it vulnerable to attack by the body's own immune system.

I purchased the ginger from farms on the Sunshine Coast and I converted it to a powder form.

I studied how the pineapple enzyme Bromelain, had been shown to inhibit cancer cell growth and how it can also induce cell apoptosis (death) in different cancers through different pathways. This enzyme is mainly found in the centre of the pineapple, which was a part I didn't normally eat, but I do now.

I researched the benefits of consuming camel milk, as I was still desperately trying to rebuild my body again. I found a camel farm at the Glasshouse Mountains on the Sunshine Coast in Queensland, and I purchased a litre of this camel milk each time it became available, which was only in the calving season.

I had now developed severe stomach issues, from my stomach lining having been destroyed, by the Opdivo and Yervoy combination, and I had been trying very hard at restoring the lining again, using natural sugar free yogurts. I purchased yogurts which contained all the necessary live cultures of Acidophilus and Bifudus. These are required by the stomach to break down the food that we eat each day. I started consuming cashew nuts, pomegranates and mangos, to name just a few, as these had also been well researched foods, and which had shown to have an ability to strengthen the body's own immune system.

I had also discovered that most of the body's immune system is housed inside the gut area itself.

I already knew that cancer thrived in acidic conditions and to reduce this, the best natural product I found to use, was the alkaline Bicarbonate of Soda, which was readily available on most supermarket shelves.

122

Each time I developed heartburn or stomach issues, I would avoid the already man-made anti-acid products, and I would add half a teaspoon of Bicarbonate of Soda powder to a small glass of water and shortly afterwards the acidity would soon disappear. I still use this technique even today, and I have shared it with many others, who have also confirmed its success for them as well.

I studied how the three pancreatic enzymes called Lipase, Protease and Amylase play a large part in the human body function of breaking down all the fats, proteins and carbohydrates from the food that we eat each day. I found that the pork pancreas was the best way to strengthen and build up these pancreatic enzymes. I contacted several butcher shops throughout South-East Queensland, trying to find a supplier of pigs' pancreas, but sadly most butchers informed me that this a part that they just throw away, as it's not used.

I then decided to look overseas, and I contacted several different companies in the USA, who explained to me that they only manufactured their pancreas supplements from pork which they sourced themselves from Southern New Zealand. They believed it was the best wild grazed supplier of pork in the world.

Too many products these days are manufactured from animals that are kept inside penned areas and not grazing wildly in open pastures. They are also being fed antibiotics, growth hormones and various other unhealthy supplements. Even a lot of our fish today is now being farmed using these products and the only fish that I trust these days are fish that I know which can't be farmed like Cod.

I have even seen where prawns which have been farmed, have developed twin heads and other malfunctions through being continuously fed antibiotics and growth hormones, to try to encourage their rapid growth.

I started having daily Coffee Enemas to detox my liver, bathing myself in water with Bicarbonate of Soda, drinking Apple Cider Vinegar that contained the essential 'mothar.' I started consuming lukewarm lemon drinks using a stainless-steel straw.

Lemon always appears acidic on the outside of the body but inside the body it changes to become more alkaline.

The reason that I used a stainless-steel straw is due to the fact, that as the lemon juice enters the body, the acidity at this stage can destroy the enamel protection on our teeth. I remembered as a boy some of the more senior people at that time always drank fresh lemon with hot water first thing in the morning, so it's an older remedy that appeared to work then and I was confident that it could work again for me. I purchased a forty-gallon container of medical food grade Hydrogen Peroxide from a company in Brisbane. I knew it was very important to source the medical grade supply instead of the regular one which is filled with toxic chemicals.

I had already started having daily baths using this peroxide in controlled amounts, to avoid it burning my body.

I studied an enzyme called Resveratrol, which is mainly found in black grape skins and red wine, and it is widely known to have a profound ability to prevent and heal many metabolic conditions including cancer cells.

It has been shown to have many protective properties, from cancer of the Prostate, Liver, Pancreas, Colon and many other organs. I continued using the natural herb again called Silybum (Milk Thistle).

I already knew that this herb had very powerful detoxifying effects on the body, and it has also been linked to the prevention and treatment of cancer cell growth of the skin. The other herb called Artichoke, has the exact same effects in helping to detoxify the liver in the human body. I knew this not only from my own experience, but I had a friend contact me regarding his liver. The doctors had told him that his liver was destroyed and that he was in a very bad way and there wasn't anything could be done now to repair it.

He started taking the Silybum (Milk Thistle) daily and he returned to the hospital several months later and the doctors was astonished at the amazing recovery he had made in the few months since his last visit.

This was enough evidence, to encourage me to continue taking it. I looked around to find a supplier of good quality Milk Thistle and I avoided the cheaper brands that normally contain inferior quality contents. I purchased a good quality water filter, fitted with a carbon insert to ensure that all the nasty chemicals are removed from my daily drinking water.

I found research that had shown were cherries had shown to help remove radiation from the body and that plums, were also tied to a thirty one percent less chance of developing any stomach cancers.

My research at this point was quite extensive, as I had no other options left available to me and I knew that the terminal condition I had, which was Stage Four Metastatic Melanoma, was regarded as being one of the worst forms of cancer for anyone to have to deal with.

Some cancers can be cut out, radiated and removed from the body, which is then monitored on a regular basis, but Metastatic Melanoma was a different form of the black beast, which travels around the body very quickly.

It uses the lymphatic system and blood vessels to spread and grow in all parts of the body, very similar to a canoeist, trying to control a canoe that is plummeting down a raging ravine. The melanoma will form a new tumour each time it stops, a bit like the canoe temporarily coming to a halt against some rock formations, along its pathway.

In September 2019 I decided to do something I had always wanted to do for a very long time.

I travelled with some friends to the Great Barrier Reef in North Queensland, and I competed in over one thousand kilometres of tarmac road rallying in a 1972 MK1 Ford Escort, which I had been restoring for some time and which I had now finished.

This was a very positive way of removing the stress of everyday cancer and an event that I thoroughly enjoyed.

It was even more special collecting the finishing medal, at the end of the week-long, event, with my navigator and friends, who were pit crewing for me the whole time.

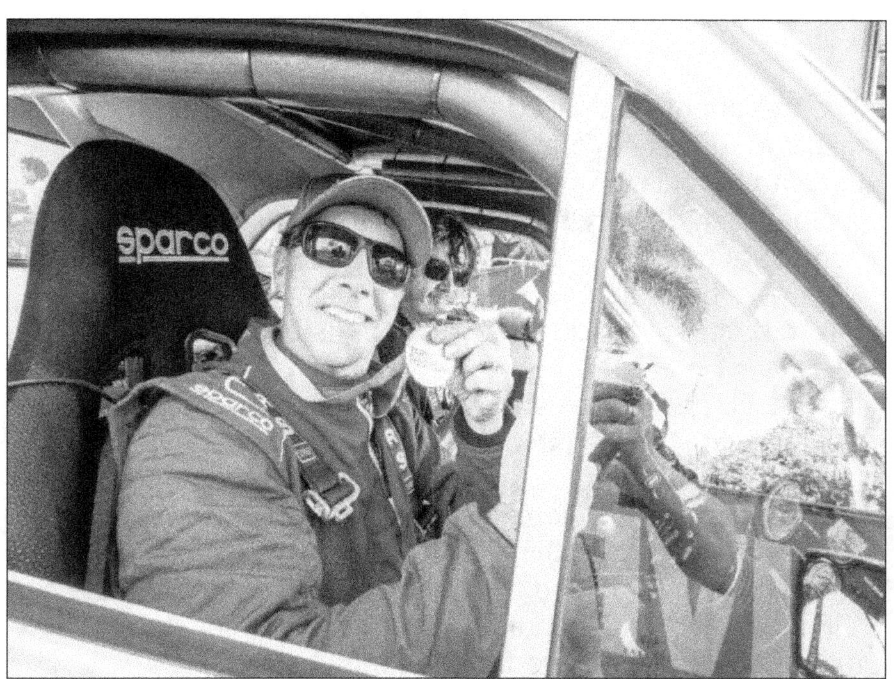

Robin at the Great Barrier Reef Car Rally in Cairns North Queensland in September 2019

For the remainder of 2019 I had managed to keep the cancer under some form of control, albeit short lived, however I believed it was better than not taking any action at all, and letting the beast take over my entire body.

I made appointments with several other oncologists in an attempt to get their help, with either the Keytruda or the Opdivo immunotherapy treatments, but they all told me the same thing each time, that nothing could save me now as my cancer was too far advanced and everything that could be done for me had already been done, and Palliative Care was now the only other option left for me, and that I should start considering it very soon.

This to me was unacceptable, and I wasn't giving in just yet. I started to research a treatment that was being widely used in Mexico.

The treatment was called Coleys Toxins, and I had discovered that several melanoma patients in the USA had used it previously, with some success. The treatment appeared to be very harsh, but anything was better than nothing at this point. It involved fitting a pic line, which runs from your heart to your arm and an intravenous drip of mixed bacteria is then used as an infusion.

It is designed to try to stimulate the body's own immune system into attacking the cancer cells and destroying the tumours. It involves the body going through a period of severe fevers and sweating, then uncontrollable chills, shakes and rigors, within a few hours of commencing the infusion. This reminded me of when I had developed the SIRS condition in December 2014, and it appeared very frightening as I continued to read about it.

In January 2020 the cancer had started on its way once again. It had spread rapidly through my body, and I was starting to develop a lot of severe pain. It appeared now to be unstoppable. The tumour on my left arm had now swollen to the size of a tennis ball, as had the one on my thigh. I was now using an arm sling to get around, which resembled walking around with a broken arm.

A friend approached me at this time regarding attending a motorsport event with him in Auckland New Zealand, as he felt that it might just help me to deal, not only with the stress I was going through, but also the severe pain that I was now in daily. It just so happened that during my research into the Coleys Toxins treatment, I discovered that the medical scientist who manufactured this treatment, was based at Auckland in New Zealand.

The lady scientist, who made this treatment for the various hospitals in Mexico that used it, had a science laboratory in Auckland.

I contacted the lady after receiving her information from another patient friend in Sydney and I travelled to Auckland in New Zealand to collect the treatment after attending the motorsport event with my friend. I had already received a letter from my own GP, explaining what the treatment was going to be used for, in case I might be denied entry at the Australian Customs carrying it back into the country.

I returned to Australia with the Coleys Toxins treatment stored inside a container in my suitcase.

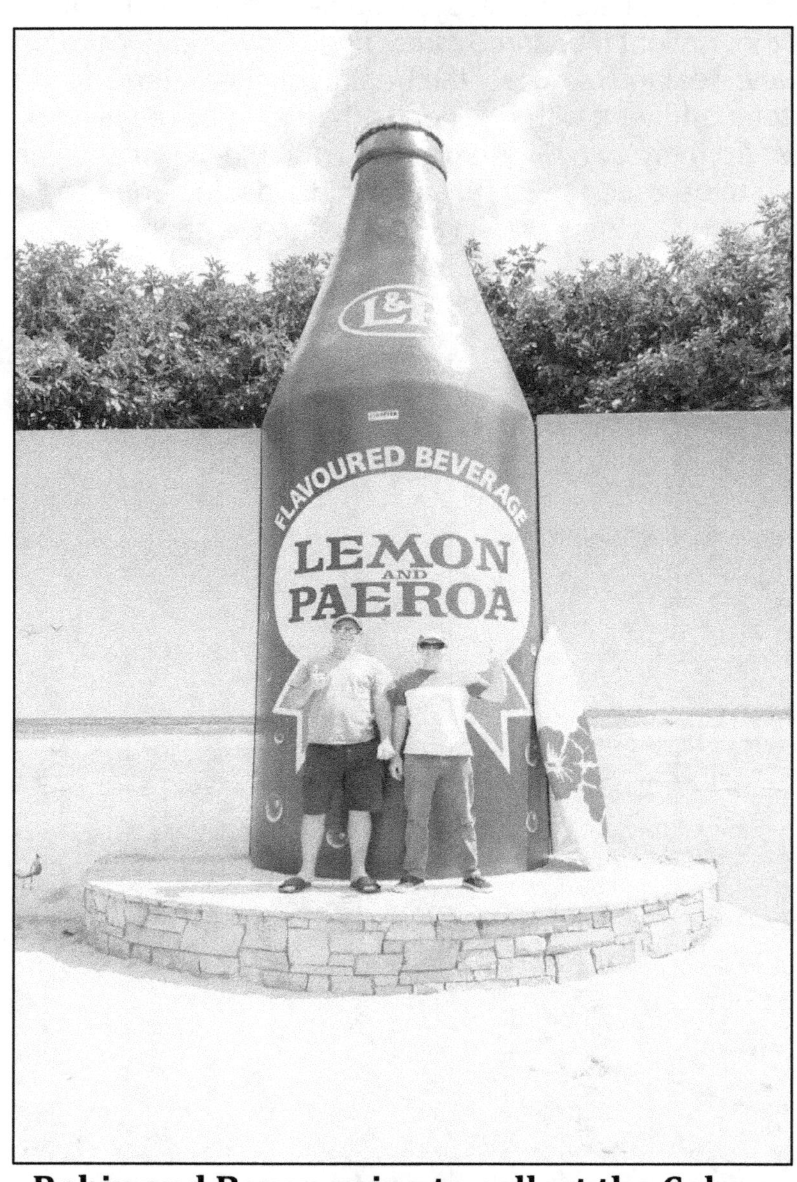

Robin and Bevan going to collect the Coleys Toxins Treatment in Auckland New Zealand

RUNNING OUT OF TIME

To allow me to continue funding the treatments which I needed to help me try to stay alive, I now had to sell the MK1 Ford Escort car, that I had recently finished building for the Great Barrier Reef rally, to a gentleman in Perth, Western Australia. Sadly, the time had now come for us to sell the very last thing we had left, which was our family home. It was now March 2020.

We had no other choice left now as our savings, and what was left of my superannuation had all been depleted from buying various treatments, in an ongoing attempt to try to stay alive. We put our house on the market for sale and we started searching for a rental property that was convenient to a nearby hospital, in case I needed access to one urgently, in the future.

After a lot of searching, we eventually managed to secure a property to rent at Currimundi, on the Sunshine Coast, which was quite close to local hospitals. It just so happened that the street was very close to our first home in Australia twenty-eight years earlier.

With the help of close friends, we moved ourselves into the rental property at Currimundi in March 2020. Not long after settling in I made an appointment to see the melanoma oncologist at the nearby local hospital, in the hope that they might be able to offer me treatment using the stand alone Opdivo immunotherapy.

I was once again refused this treatment, and I was told that 'in their opinion' due, to the fact that I had 'failed' with the previous PDL-1 treatment of Keytruda (Pembolizumab), that the Opdivo treatment would not work for me either. Once again this was totally wrong, as you will find out soon, that it was the Keytruda treatment that I was wrongly taken off in 2017 that helped to save my life in the end.

The Keytruda and the Opdivo are very similar treatments, except that they are both manufactured by two different pharmaceutical companies. I was told if I really wanted the treatment, then I would have to purchase it, myself at a cost of six thousand dollars every three weeks. I begged to be considered for the treatment, which was now being used daily in all the public hospitals in Australia, by other public patients.

I told them yet again, that I was very confident from my own research, and from the recent test results that I had received from both the laboratories in Germany and Arizona, that it could work in my favour to fight my cancer. I showed the oncologists the test results from Germany and Arizona, but they were ignored and some even referred to them as being pure rubbish and just another scam that I must have been caught up in.

So much I thought for your views and opinions on genetic testing, which I was very confident was what was needed in all cancer cases these days, instead of just trying to treat people with a one glove fits all approach and only using guess work. Everybody is different and we all respond in different ways. No DNA is identical.

It was now totally impossible for me to find the money I needed to fund this treatment on my own, as it amounted to thousands of dollars each week.

This cost was also going to be in addition to our normal weekly six hundred dollars rent payment, food, phone and every other essential service that we had to pay, for our everyday living needs.

I asked once again if it would be possible to be granted the treatment compassionately from the pharmaceutical supplier, as I was aware of other patients being able to obtain their treatments this way. I was told that it could not be provided to me compassionately as they had already requested this from the pharmaceutical companies on my behalf. I also knew from before, that both companies had never heard from them from any of these oncologists.

In the rental accommodation I decided, that for me to keep trying to fight my cancer, I would have no other option at this stage but to start treating myself in the bedroom, come makeshift hospital ward, with the Coleys Toxins therapy, that I had brought back with me from New Zealand in January.

The issue I was now faced with was trying to find, either a doctor or a surgeon who specialised in Cardiac surgery, who would be able to fit the pic lines which I needed, running from my arm to my heart. I made several phone calls before I finally found a cardiologist, who was based at the Buderim private hospital on the Sunshine Coast, and who agreed to fit the Pic lines into my arm, which would then run directly to my heart. The pic line is where the daily infusions would then be connected to, for the drip feed to my body.

Again, with not having any private health hospital cover, the cost of having the surgery completed, theatre hire, hospital costs and the anaesthetist amounted to five thousand dollars.

The more I thought about the totally unnecessary chemotherapy that I had been given, that started all this in the first place, the more upset I was starting to become. I had endured so much pain, stress, financial burden and the ongoing illness because of unnecessary chemical poisoning from a totally ridiculous medical decision. I attended the hospital on the prearranged day for the pic line procedure. As I had already done many times before, I changed into my theatre gown before being prepared for the surgery by the anaesthetist. I had the operation carried out and I left the hospital later that same day with the two pic line toggles hanging out of my arm. I was informed that these two toggles attached to the pic line would require cleaning each week by professional nurses, due to the fact, that the line was running directly to my heart.

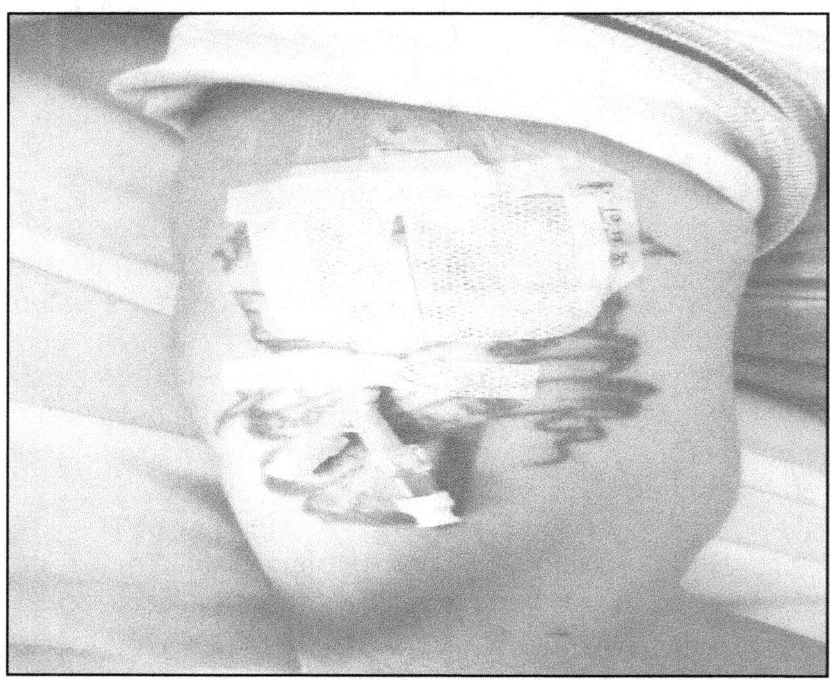

Pic Line fitted into Robin's arm going directly to his heart, for the Coleys Toxins infusions

I returned home again with the pic line now inserted into my arm and leading directly to my heart. I had already contacted my GP, regarding having some nurses call at my house each week to clean the toggles hanging from the line, that would require regular maintenance. Over the next two days the pic line started to leak a lot of blood, so I had to return to the clinic once again to have this attended to. After another few days it finally sealed itself and I stopped bleeding.

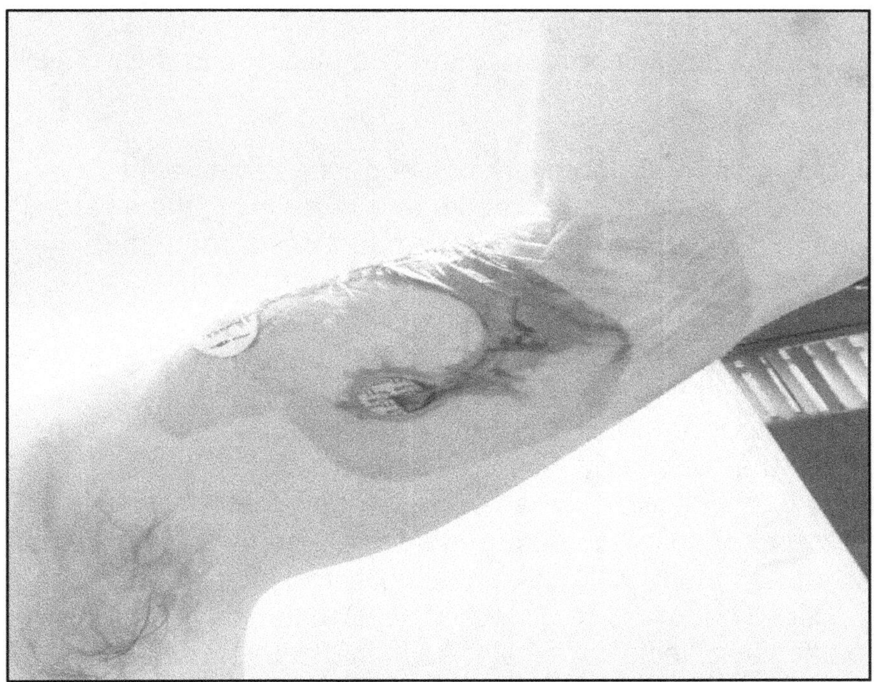

The Pic Line starting to leak my blood

I contacted the Blue Nurses in Queensland, and they kindly agreed to visit me once a week at my rental accommodation, to clean both lines and to change the drip feed attachment toggles. As these were running straight to my heart, regular maintenance was extremely important.

The Blue nurses left me a list of what I would require each week for them to carry out their work and I ordered the intravenous Saline bags, intravenous tubes, surgical gloves, fluid rate adjusters, cleaning wipes, in fact everything that I would require to commence my own treatment infusions in a home surgery environment.

I purchased a hat stand frame to hang the infusion bags from, an inflatable bed which I could lie on and everything that I would need to convert a normal bedroom into a hospital ward, to commence treating myself with the Coleys Toxins.

I told my wife and some friends about the treatment that I was soon about to commence, and like myself, they were all deeply concerned, as the vast amount of research had shown that some patients had died from using it.

My wife approached my own GP about her concerns, and he told her that he was also very worried about it, however it was entirely up to Robin, but if he didn't try something very soon, the melanoma would kill him anyway as he was in a very bad way at this time. I already knew from my own research both online and from several phone conversations that I had made with various doctors, including some in the Mexican hospitals, to expect chills, sweats, shivering and other side effects once I started to infuse the treatment directly into my body.

I was also told to avoid trying to bring my body out of these various conditions, as by doing so it would affect the outcome of the treatment, that I had just administered to myself.

The advice I was given, was that when the shakes and chills get too severe, then place a blanket over my body and avoid consuming cold drinks, but instead sip occasionally on vitamin drinks, similar to a Berocca.

I decided that I would commence this treatment the following week. The therapy information which had been supplied with the Coleys Toxins, was very clear and precise, that over the duration of the six-week daily programme, the bacteria infusion should only be commenced very slowly, with a certain milligram strength each day.

This was mixed with the saline in the infusion bag, as my body needed time to be able to deal slowly, with the effects of the bacteria triggering the anticipated immune system response. I knew that if I got this wrong at the very beginning, that it would have very serious consequences for my life.

A serious immune response early in the treatment would be life threatening, and very similar to the near-death SIRS (Severe Immune Response Syndrome) that I had previously suffered in December 2014, from the targeted therapy.

After I had prepared the first mix of saline and Coleys Toxins together in the infusion bag, I then attached it to the hat stand I had previously purchased, which would then act as a drip feed surgery stand. My heart was pounding at this time, and I had already set up a blood pressure monitor next to my inflatable bed and I had wrapped it around my right arm.

This way I would then be able to monitor my blood pressure during the anticipated side effects episodes, and chart it each day, to help me keep a recorded system, that I could refer to later, if I needed to.

This was to collect information on when the shakes and chills started and finished each day, as well as my blood pressure rate at the same time as well.

I attached the drip feed line to the saline bag and ensured that the line had the necessary fluid rate control switch attached to it, which would then allow me to regulate the rate at which the drip would be entering into my body through my right arm. I then lay down on the inflatable bed and attached the tube to the pic line which was hanging out of my arm and leading directly to my heart.

As soon as I started the fluid flow, I noticed a very large air bubble advancing towards my arm inside the intravenous line. This frightened me, as I knew that large air bubbles could cause issues. I grabbed the infusion line and kinked it over to stop the fluid reaching the entrance to the pic line.

I disconnected the line, and I started it again a second time. Eventually over the next few weeks I had managed to become an expert with these intravenous supply lines.

I then lay on the inflatable bed awaiting the anticipated first side effects to begin. After the first hour I began to feel the cold chills and slight shaking which very soon became uncontrollable shaking. I was shaking so violently that the whole airbed was literally moving around the bedroom floor, like a floating hovercraft.

It was a very frightening moment and my wife at this point asked me did I want an ambulance called, to which I replied "No, just let it run its course." I pulled the woollen blanket up around my neck and I prayed that I would survive this very serious condition that was now happening to me.

Finally, after approximately half an hour of violent shaking it stopped, and the chills then turned to hot sweaty fevers. I was then able to remove the blanket which I had earlier pulled up over myself during the chill period and I started sipping the Vitamin B fluid, which I had already prepared earlier, before I started the infusion. I had survived the first treatment and I was very thankful indeed. I continued this daily treatment for six weeks and the weekly home visits from the Blue Nurses managed to keep my pic lines safe and clean, from each of the visits they made. The nurses who attended to me at the rental property were extremely helpful, and it was always nice to see them coming, and to have a friendly chat with them.

During this period, I decided that in order to help me keep my sanity that I would work on another old car project. Each afternoon once I had finished my treatment and I felt fully recovered, I travelled to my friend's property at Glenview, on the Sunshine Coast and I worked on restoring an old Ford Anglia car.

I had to be extremely careful during the cutting, welding and grinding processes as I had to protect the two pic line toggles that were still hanging out of my arm. I purchased an old welder's leather jacket, and I secured some extra straps around my arm for added protection from the sparks and metal grinding that occurred whilst doing this work.

After six weeks I went back to the hospital for another whole-body PET scan. Sadly, this scan showed that the treatment that I had hoped would bring me the most success had regrettably not brought me any success at all, and the cancer was now continuing to spread rapidly throughout my body. The six weeks of daily suffering and torment had all been in vain, but at least I had tried once again.

A day that I will always remember from this period when I managed to have some humour, was one afternoon when I returned to the rental accommodation from my friend's property. After working on my car restoration project I opened the rear lid top of my vehicle to discover that a black chicken had managed to jump onboard in a failed escape attempt from my friend's property.

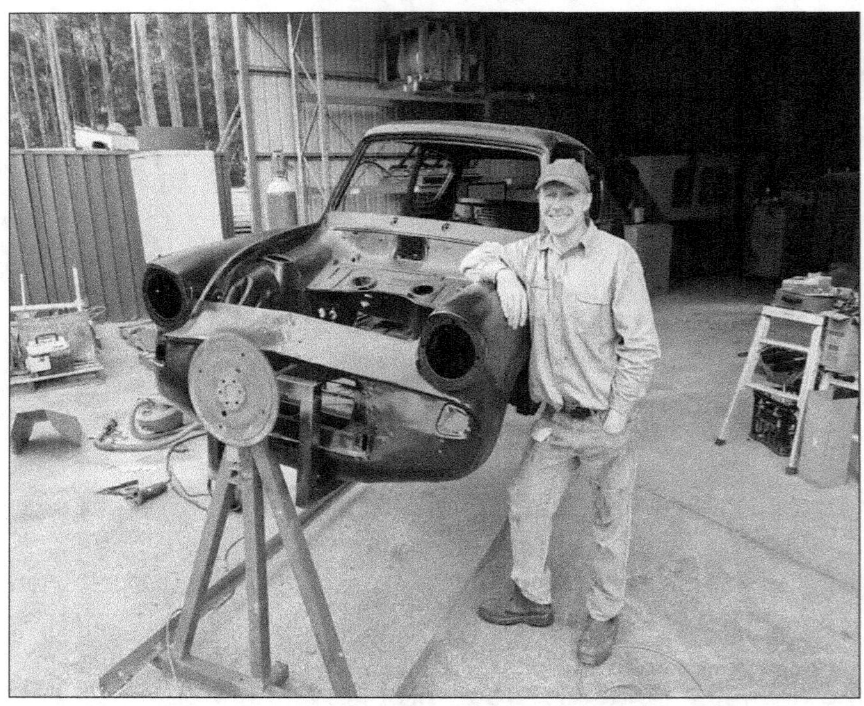

Robin working on his Anglia car restoration

I returned the chicken back to the property an hour later. Apparently, this same black chicken had already made several previous failed attempts to escape from the property.

After I decided to cease the Coleys Toxins, I made another appointment to see the cardiologist at Buderim to have the pic line removed from my arm.

He was able to carry out this procedure in his own clinic and I was glad to have it finally removed from my arm.

With no success now either, from using the Coleys Toxins therapy, I was again extremely disappointed. I didn't really have any choices left now with any further treatment options. Up to this stage all my tumours had been internal cancers, but now the beast was becoming very much more aggressive, and several new tumours had suddenly started to appear externally.

I had developed tumours on the side of my skull above my right ear, on my forehead, neck, chest, and under both my arm pits. The black beast was now furiously trying to take over my body in another attempt to kill me, and once again, I was searching frantically to find any other sort of help that I could.

I researched where a product called Gossypin, had been successful in treating melanoma cancer. It's a product made from both Hibiscus and Cotton flowers. I ordered a large supply of this supplement from the USA, but again sadly I could not find any success from using it and I didn't order any more. I then discovered a dog worming product called Fenbendazole, as some people had claimed it had been successful in helping them with their cancers. I ordered a supply of these capsules from the US and despite taking them each day, I also found after a few months, that they too also appeared to be ineffective, as new tumours kept showing up at various locations around my body.

Sadly, during this period as others were also beginning to find out about this product, the price of these worming capsules from most of the veterinary clinics across the USA had increased in cost from five US dollars each to thirty US dollars per capsule.

141

I returned once more to the hospital, and I was referred to their radiation department instead. Here, I was told the same as I had already been told before, that nothing can save you now and the only thing we can offer you for your pain relief is radiation.

I was very nervous again as even though the Gamma Knife radiation had been very successful treating my previous brain tumours, I was concerned now, that in the event of widespread whole-body radiation, that the explosive consequences of trying to destroy these tumours might result in the cancer cells spreading the cancer further throughout my body, as my research had shown that this can happen very quickly. I was in a lot of extreme pain at this time, and I very reluctantly agreed to have the radiation therapy carried out, as all the pain killers I was being prescribed, were causing me very severe constipation, which is a known side effect of taking pain killers on a regular basis.

The following week I went to the hospital and a foam frame was formed to my own body's shape, which was then set up as a bed frame. This was to be the frame that I would be strapped to each day, for each radiation procedure over the next few weeks. Both my arms and chest were tattooed with black ink marks, which would be used as alignment markers for the radiation machine.

These markers would be used to help identify where the radiation would be required to strike the various cancer tumour sites accurately, that had already been identified in the CT scans taken the week before.

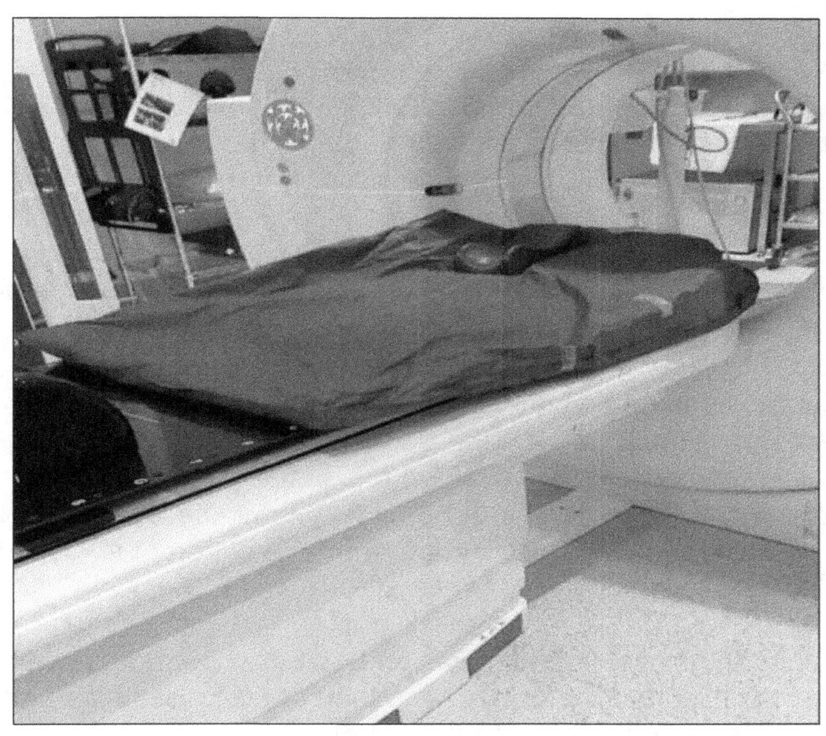

The moulded Radiation Body Bed Frame

For the next 6 weeks I was attached each day to a radiation machine. My body was radiated in so many places, starting with the tumour on my forehead and neck, right down to my feet. I had now developed a large tumour on my back which was the size of a pineapple, and various other tumours had now appeared around my shoulder area, which were horrendously sore. After the six weeks was finished, I went back to the hospital for further scans to see if this radiation therapy had shown any success in destroying the tumours.

The scans showed that the radiation had achieved absolutely nothing and all I had ended up with was more painful burns everywhere on my body. The radiation specialist at the hospital then told me later, that most times the radiation doesn't work for melanoma cancers.

143

I wondered why I wasn't told this before the treatment commenced, instead of being told this afterwards, when it was all over. I could have then made my own informed decision, as to whether, or not I would have decided to proceed with it or not.

I was in a lot of pain now, and I had my own doctor prescribe me more painkillers and patches. I didn't want to have to resort to this, but sadly I now **knew that** I had no other choice, as the pain was becoming very extreme. The tumour around my shoulder and the large tumour on my back were now unbearably sore. I decided to consult with a very well-known and respected surgeon on the Sunshine Coast to see if he could remove these tumours, or even attempt to dissect a portion of them, to try to relieve my pain.

During this consultation, I was told that the operations would be too difficult to perform, due to their specific locations and there was also too big an element of risk involved.

The surgeon apologised that he couldn't help me any further and wished me luck. At this point I knew that I was going to really need to have a lot of luck, if I was going to be able to continue my fight with this cancerous monster.

Another new tumour had appeared on the left side of my face beside my left ear. I decided to travel to Brisbane and to discuss its possible removal with a private surgeon at his Ear, Nose and Throat clinic in the Spring Hill district, as my previous Ear, Nose and Throat specialist, had now retired from his practice. I had researched this surgeon, and from the feedback and reviews he had received, I felt quite comfortable requesting his help. Unfortunately, as my face had already been cut open at that same site in the previous unnecessary surgery a year earlier, he felt that it would now be impossible to re-open it there once again.

He informed me that this could cause me very serious complications, similar to those that I might have developed, had I allowed the first surgeon to operate there, with the anticipated nerve, eye and mouth permanent damage, which would have resulted. I also decided to ask him during this consultation if he could remove the tumour that had suddenly appeared on my forehead and the one on my neck. He said that for this type of surgery his brother would be the best person to carry it out, as his speciality was cosmetic surgery. He kindly gave me a reference to his brother, who also had his own private clinic in Albion, another nearby suburb of Brisbane. I thanked him for his help and I left the clinic.

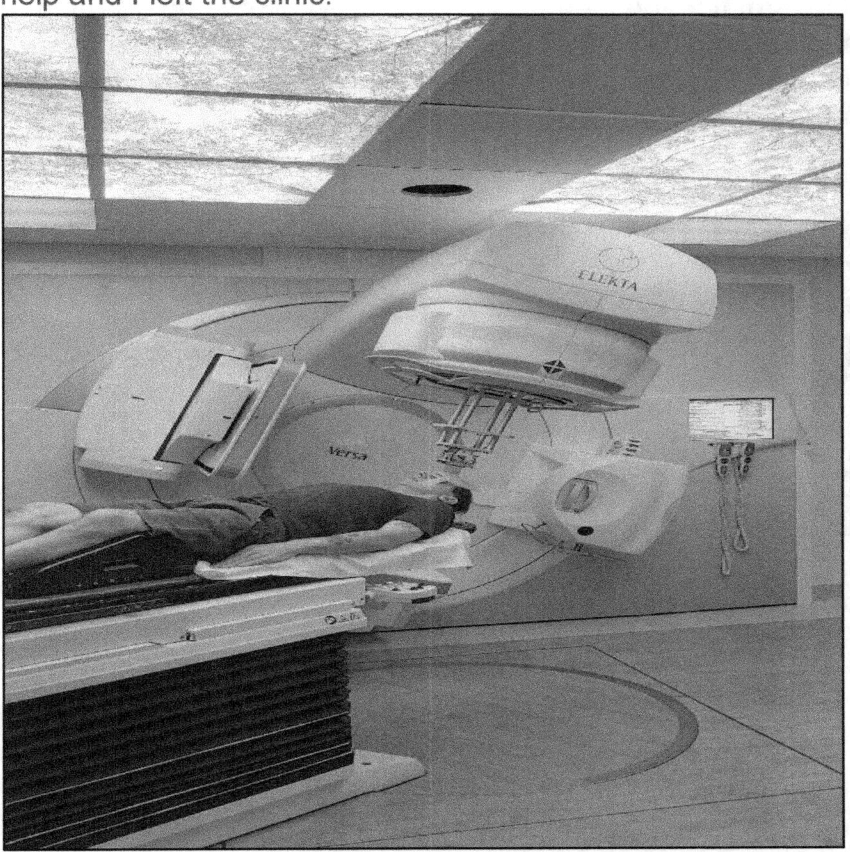

The failed radiation on the Forehead Tumour

145

THE CUTTING BEGINS AND ALMOST THE END

A few weeks later I travelled back to Brisbane, for a meeting with the new surgeon in Albion. He discussed the procedure he would use, regarding the removal of several of the tumours from both my neck, including the tumour I now had on my forehead, and I agreed to trust his skills to proceed with the removal of these melanoma tumours. A date was set, and I returned once again in a few weeks' time. At this appointment he removed both the tumours under local anaesthetic, and I left his clinic stitched across my forehead and neck like a badly bruised boxer, and less another three thousand dollars. Several weeks later I had the stitches removed by a practice nurse on the Sunshine Coast. I was content with the outcome, and over the next few weeks the wounds slowly began to heal once again.

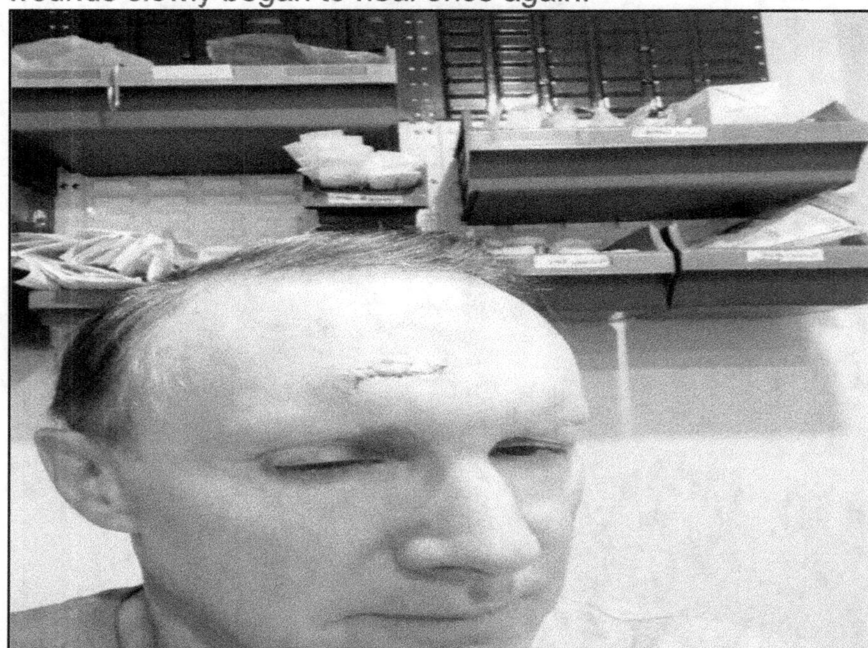

Surgical Forehead Tumour removal operation

Sadly, this was only to be the beginning of many more surgical procedures, I had to request his help with, in my continued struggle with this beast inside me, that seemed determined to keep trying to destroy me quickly. I continued with my daily study, and I found out that recent studies had clearly proven that cancer patients should avoid using certain cooking oils. The research had shown that Sunflower oil, Peanut oil and Canola oil, all oxidise once they are inside the human body, and they can then actually promote further cancer growth and spread. I started to restrict my use of cooking oil to only using a good quality Virgin Oil instead. I rarely consumed peanuts, but I had also found research that had shown were the consumption of peanuts, was indeed also linked to the spread of existing cancer and were to be avoided by people with cancer.

The water purification system I had previously purchased was shown to remove fluoride from the water, as well as all the other 'nasties' that we want to try to avoid drinking each day. When I had attended the cancer clinic in Berlin, the doctor there told me that fluoride had been banned from use in Germany many years earlier, due to information that was received, confirming that it was well known to calcify the pineal gland inside the body. This is the gland that secretes Melatonin, the body's natural sleep hormone. It has been known to calcify much quicker in elderly people, which means that it can become much more difficult for them to sleep later in life, so removing the fluoride early on in life was quite important. It is also regularly used by dentists after completing dental procedures, so I avoided this as well on each of my dental appointments.

I discovered through my dental research, that the amalgam (grey coloured) fillings that are used daily in dental procedures, are also quite dangerous for cancer patients.

This is due to the fact, that the amalgam fillings themselves contain mercury, and this is the reason why people can sometimes notice a strange metallic taste in their mouth. This taste occurs as a result of the mercury leakage from the amalgam fillings. I decided to have all my existing amalgam fillings removed and replaced as further protection. I found a naturopathic dentist at Maroochydore on the Sunshine Coast, who regularly carried out this procedure. This was a rather difficult process, as all the existing fillings had to broke up first, in order to be removed. There was also an even greater risk at this point, that some of the debris from the amalgam fillings might be swallowed in the body, causing even greater harm. It was a process that took quite a few dental appointments and another cost of six thousand dollars, until the entire removal process was complete.

I remembered back to when I was a young child, the thermometer that the doctors and nurses used to use to take your body's temperature with, when you were sick or had developed a fever. The glass one that was placed under your tongue was filled with mercury. I can only but think back now of how dangerous that must have been, when considering it could very easily have been broken by someone in a wrongful bite. Thankfully modern-day equipment now used in all the hospitals and clinics to take temperature readings, is much more sophisticated and less dangerous than it was back then in that period.

With no treatment options available to me now whatsoever, I was really struggling to find a way to try to stop this vicious cancer from continuing to spread itself throughout my body.

New tumours had suddenly appeared under both my arm pits, on my chest and on the side of my scalp above my ear.

This was in addition to the huge tumours that I already had on my back, and the large one on my shoulder region, that none of the surgeons would attempt to operate on.

I still had the massive tumour on my thigh, and on my left arm. Life was becoming more and more intolerable each day and trying to sleep with so many tumours, was now virtually impossible.

I reluctantly agreed to start attending the Sunshine Coast Palliative Care Centre in Caloundra at this time, for more pain relief. Sadly, I had no other options left and the painkillers were being increased every few days. I was now taking massive amounts of Targin and Oxycodone, just to name a few. Although these did help me to mask the pain for a short period, they didn't really help me either, as painkillers are well known for developing constipation, and I already had a large tumour which was partially blocking my bowel.

The radiation treatment had not helped me at all in any way, and in fact the way that my cancer was now spreading throughout my entire body like a wildfire, indicated, that the radiation had done me more harm than it had done me good, and I believe that as a result of receiving it in the first place, that it had indeed instigated the swift progression of my cancer.

It was now the last week of August 2020. The Palliative Care doctor decided that I should have a CT scan of my abdominal region, due to the severe and uncontrollable pain that I was now suffering.

The scan showed that I now had over thirty new tumours in my abdominal region alone, some of which were up to fifteen millimetres in size.

The huge tumour on my chest wall, which was the size of a
tennis ball, was now measuring eleven centimetres by three
centimetres, a mass of thirty-three centimetres. This tumour
was still less than half the size of the one I already had on
my lower back, which now resembled a rugby ball
measuring twelve centimetres by six centimetres, a mass of
almost seventy-two centimetres. The tumour on my left
shoulder and back shoulder region was now measuring nine
centimetres by five centimetres, a mass of forty-five
centimetres. It was massive and it felt like I was constantly
carrying a backpack around with me, twenty-four hours a
day. It was virtually impossible to sleep at any time, and I
was using a variety of different types of heat and cool packs,
as well as deep heat creams. It was now October 2020. The
tumour, which was growing on the side of my scalp, I
decided now that I would try different ways to remove it
myself. I tried DMSO liquid mixed with MSM and Bicarbonate potion. I even tried injecting into it myself with
various solutions as well as attempting to cut part of it way
with a blade.

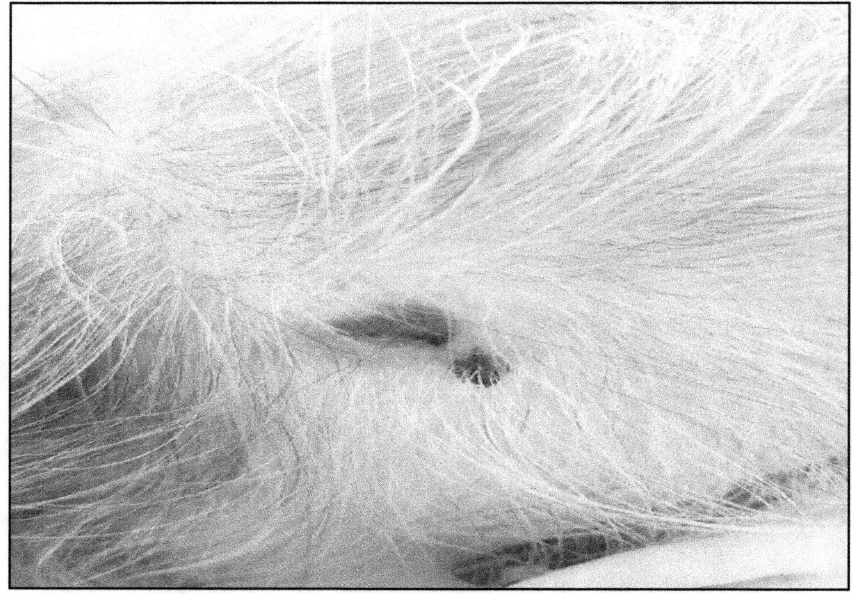

The large Tumour that appeared on the scalp

At this time, I had been researching Folistatin, and I ordered this from the UK to see if it could help me in any way to destroy the tumour. I asked my GP for a prescription, as this was required to be able to purchase it. I also needed it to be able to allow access through Australian Customs, in case the treatment might be treated as a steroid of some type, and it might be denied entry into the country.

The Folistatin vials arrived quickly, and I immediately started to inject the solution directly into the tumour for a week, and although it did help to remove a portion of the tumour, which resulted in a large hole appearing in my scalp, sadly it wasn't enough to remove it entirely, as the tumour was very deep and large.

I decided then that the only way to remove this tumour, including the other small tumours on my chest, and the ones that had suddenly appeared under my arms, would be once again, to have them surgically removed under the surgeon's scalpel. I made another private appointment with the same surgeon at Albion in Brisbane, and on the same day I attended his practice, he was able to remove all four tumours at once, under a local anaesthetic procedure.

The pain from the huge tumours on my back and shoulder had now become unbearable, and I went to the Emergency Department of the local hospital on several occasions to try to see what they could do to help me. Once again, I requested if they could even remove the tumour from my left arm, as I was now permanently using a sling and the Blue nurses were attending the house each week with pain killing patches, which were then strapped around my arm.

I decided to request a referral to the orthopaedic department of another hospital on the south side of Brisbane, for yet another second opinion on trying to remove this tumour.

The surgical team at the hospital examined the scans they had now received. After reviewing the scans of the tumour, which had now progressed rapidly throughout the large network of veins, nerves and arteries, it was decided that the complications that could result from carrying out any form of surgical removal, would be too dangerous. They also said that there was a very high degree of risk involved that could result in me losing my arm completely.

I had finally reached a stage in my struggle with this beast where I thought it wasn't worth trying to continue to keep fighting it. I had fought it as hard as I possibly could, however I couldn't see any way forward out of this awful situation. I started to investigate euthanasia both here in Australia and in Switzerland. I discussed it with my family, who fully understood my present situation and how rapid the progression of this disease now was.

Euthanasia had not been made legal in Queensland at this time, but it was available in most others Australian States. My family said they would support me if I wanted to travel to Switzerland, and they would accompany me there to say my final goodbyes to them all. I gave this some very deep consideration, but I decided not to go ahead with it for various reasons including the fact that we simply could not afford the trip either, as our funds were almost depleted. I knew that my chances of staying alive much longer were becoming very slim each day, and the suffering was becoming more and more intolerable to bear.

I got up out of bed one morning, where I was now spending most of my time surrounded by painkillers, heat packs, ice packs, in fact anything that might just help to ease my pain. I left the house where we were still renting at this time, and I got into my vehicle, and drove to a nearby hardware store.

I walked into the plumbing section of the store where I purchased some hose pipe, which I knew I could fit to the exhaust pipe of my vehicle. I picked a length of flexible hose which would be long enough to reach from the back of my vehicle's exhaust pipe to the driver's side window. I then purchased a pillow and a roll of duct tape, which I would also use to seal the window effectively. I placed these into the back of my vehicle, and I drove back to the rental property.

This was my decision and my decision alone. I hadn't discussed it with anyone else at this time. The next issue I had was to select somewhere to bring this constant pain and suffering, finally to an end. Not just for me, but also for my family, who had been suffering my torment for long enough as well.

After having lived on the Sunshine Coast in Queensland for many years, I had become very familiar with most of the local forests and their inroads and pathways. I selected an old road between Caloundra and Landsborough to bring this daily suffering to an end. A few days later I got up once again at first light and I left the rental accommodation where we were still staying at this time through the rear side door, so as not to awaken anyone else in the house and I headed off, on this my own personal mission.

As I travelled along the road, I had many things running through my head. I pulled off the main road to the location where I had selected to end this suffering.

I started to write a final letter which I would then leave on top of the dash in my vehicle. I knew that occasionally other traffic used this same road daily, so it would only be a matter of time before I would be discovered.

153

I sat in the vehicle for a few minutes as I still had the hose pipe in the rear tray at this stage. I was still unsure if this was the way I was to finally depart Gods earth. After a few minutes I decided that no, this was a coward's way out and it wasn't the way I was meant to depart. Even though I was suffering so much pain at this time, both physically and emotionally, it wasn't the way I was meant to go. I started up my vehicle and turned around from the side road where I had parked up and I drove back to the rental accommodation. I opened the rear tray of my vehicle, and I took out the roll of hose pipe. I placed it into the wheelie bin nearby. I went back into the house as nobody was awake yet, and I climbed back into bed. I never mentioned to anyone about what had just taken place.

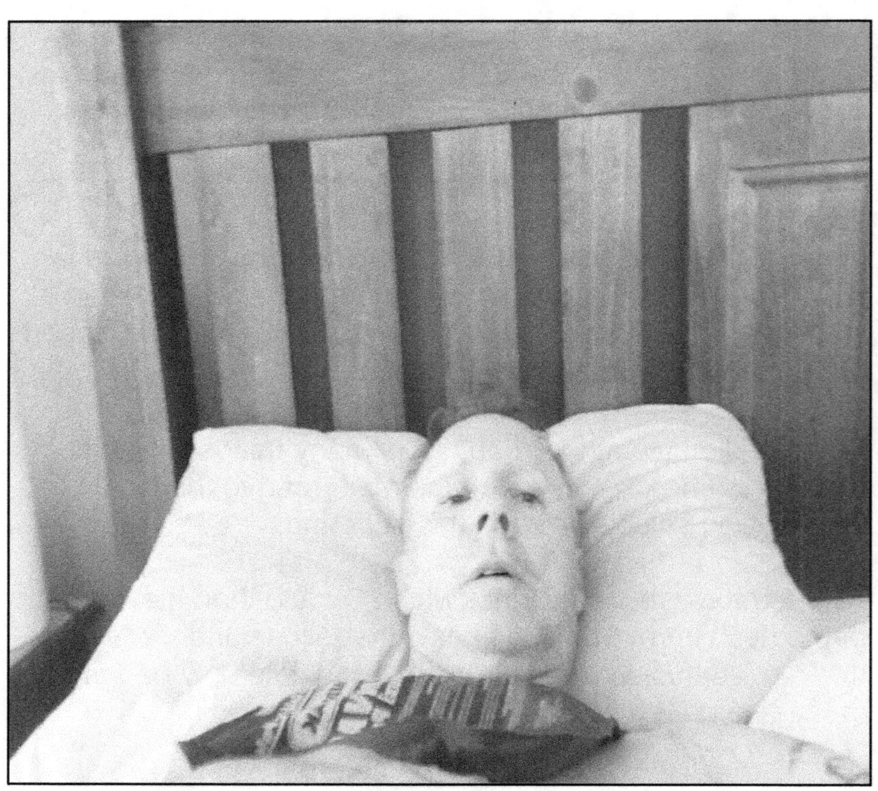

Very close to the final chapter at this stage

The cancer was now rapidly running rampant and out of control.

New tumours had appeared inside my body everywhere and this included my bowel, which was now partly blocked, and I was having to use a tube and an enema bag as a toilet method as a large tumour had formed between by hips at my anus, which was making it impossible to sit anywhere.

I purchased several doughnut-style cushions as this was the only way I could rest in a chair, or lay on a bed, or even to attempt to sit in a car seat, without enduring excruciating pain.

I decided as I was now unable to get any further appointments with any hospital oncologists, I would try to email them personally, begging for their help, as I knew that my time was becoming very short with no hospital treatment now for almost three years.

I emailed three oncologists that I had previously met, but it was without any success each time. One in fact told me 'Please stop bothering me,' and another oncologist replied by telling me that nothing could save me now, as I had previously failed all the treatments that were available to me and no anti-PD1 (immunotherapy) would work for me now, as it was impossible and a waste of time even trying it. They even recited the medical Hippocratic Oath to me in which they all swear a promise to do no harm to a patient.

I replied to this email by stating, that after almost three years without any form of cancer fighting treatment of any type, even after my own genetic testing had been completed in laboratories in both Germany, and Phoenix Arizona in the USA had all proven that I would respond to either Opdivo or Keytruda, was in fact doing me harm.

I received another reply again, in which I was told that they fully understood the Hippocratic Oath, so in other words, stop bothering me.

I was clearly wasting my time here with this oncologist as it was going nowhere, I was achieving absolutely nothing, and it appeared to me as being totally hypocritical.

I decided to try to request help from both my local Member of Parliament, and from my Federal Member of Parliament. I wrote personal letters to both MPs but sadly their responses offered me no help whatsoever, as I pleaded to be given the opportunity to save my own life, which was sadly rapidly diminishing. I decided to contact the Melanoma Institute in Sydney to try to find some help from them regarding any impending clinical trials that I might be able to participate in. Unfortunately, as I had so many brain tumours previously, this then apparently eliminated me from being able to qualify for any other up and coming future clinical cancer trials. They did suggest however, that I should contact an oncologist who practiced on the Gold Coast in Queensland, regarding a melanoma trial that had just finished called the LEAP 004 trial.

This trial had been shown to produce some excellent results, using Keytruda immunotherapy, which was the very first treatment I had originally selected for myself at the beginning and the one which I was later taken off by an oncologist at the hospital in Brisbane, as they (very wrongly) told me that it wasn't working for me. The other treatment was called Lenvatinib. I thanked them very much indeed for informing me of this trial and for their help, which I appreciated very much and which I would now follow up.

delay but I have been on leave and only back <u>today</u>.
- I honestly feel for you right now and really would love
to offer you as much hope as possible but I can not
give you false hope and am bound by oath to first do no
harm. The reason why I will not prescribe the
Nivolumab however is because your disease
progressed despite you being given many months of a
course of anti-PD1 previously. There is no chance the
cancer would now respond to a further course of anti-
PD1.

An Oncologist's reply, saying that there is now no chance that any immunotherapy treatment would save me. Don't always believe what you are being told. I am the living proof of this.

FINALLY HOPE FROM DARKNESS

I immediately had a feeling that this was a treatment that could work for me again this time around. I didn't find out until much later, that the Keytruda treatment would have continued to work for me previously all along, and that I should never have been taken off it in the very first place. This was another shocking case of medical negligence, that destroyed me, financially, physically and emotionally.

I contacted the Health Care provider on the Gold Coast in Queensland, to request an appointment to meet with this oncologist. I knew now that I was in a very serious health position, and I probably wasn't going to be able to reach Christmas unless I tried something immediately. My problem at this stage was that the cost of the treatment, which I would have to fund again myself, was totally prohibitive. The Keytruda alone was six thousand dollars every three weeks and the Lenvatinib was four thousand dollars. It was going to be totally impossible for me to find ten thousand dollars every three weeks, on top of our weekly rent and everything else that we had to pay for, as part of our daily living expenses.

We still had minimal resources left from selling our own home, as we were now sadly confined to only being able to live in rental accommodation, and the cost to date of the treatments I had been forced to purchase was in excess of five hundred thousand dollars.

Even if the treatment did start to show me any signs of success, which I believed it would, I didn't know how much longer I would be able to continue purchasing it.

On top of the treatment costs, there were also the associated costs of each clinic visit, the doctor's consultation fee, the hospital bed, the nurses, the infusion materials, the travel to the Gold Coast, toll road charges. All these costs were in addition to the initial cost of the treatment itself. These additional fees I later calculated at six hundred dollars for each clinic appointment, bringing the total cost of each visit to the clinic every three weeks to six thousand six hundred dollars, for just the Keytruda alone.

The oncologist confirmed an appointment with me by email, however he requested that before he could meet up with me to discuss my current situation, I would first be required to have a whole-body PET scan conducted, which would reveal the full extent of the cancer devastation that was going on inside my body at that time. A scan was subsequently arranged at a hospital in Buderim on the Sunshine Coast for the 10th of November 2020.

I attended the hospital appointment on this day as planned. Shortly after arrival it was discovered that there was a big problem trying to insert the cannula injection needle into my veins, for the glucose to be infused. My veins had become so weak from all the abuse they had received over the past ten years. Finally, after several attempts by many different nurses, a doctor was finally called into the treatment room and a portable ultrasound device was obtained from a different hospital department.

After a few minutes of using this device, a vein was finally found, into which the cannula was inserted for the infusion to begin.

As is customary with these PET scans I then had to wait in the room for an hour, without any form of body movement whatsoever, whilst the glucose infusion was distributed around my entire body, throughout my network of veins.

After an hour, I was then taken out of the room and walked down the corridor, to the where the PET scanning device was located. This is the machine, which would be used to take images of where the cancer could be seen to be feeding on the glucose infusion. I was then placed into the imaging machine, and this was where I would remain, for the next forty-five minutes duration, in order to complete the necessary scanning procedures.

After a few days the report was finalised. It was a horrific finding. The report confirmed that I was in an extremely bad way. I had approximately fifteen tumours in my brain alone and dozens all around my body, which were in addition to the one's that I was already aware off. I had in total approximately ninety tumours of all various shapes and sizes throughout my entire body. The report stated that I had extensive tumours stretching from my head, right down to the calves on the back of my legs.

Now that we had a finalised report completed, I was able to confirm an appointment with the oncologist on the Gold Coast, for early December 2020. As I was now very much aware of the mass of tumours in my brain, I fully understood the severity of the situation and it was indeed, very dire.

Up to this stage I had also managed to form a close relationship with the brain radiation specialist at a south Brisbane hospital. He was the doctor who had previously carried out my Targeted Gamma Knife radiation in March 2017. He is a specialist whom I respect, and I have total confidence in.

From 2017, he has arranged for me to have regular brain scans carried out every three months, to help monitor any cancer activity in my brain.

Sadly, however these fifteen new tumours had suddenly appeared since my last hospital MRI scan, which once again confirmed to me, just how quickly this disease can take over your entire body in such a very short time. I also knew that he worked privately with another large cancer group in Queensland. I decided to contact him immediately and an appointment was arranged at the private clinic, where he also practiced.

At this appointment I explained to him about my latest crisis situation. I knew if I waited to get an appointment at the public hospital that I probably wouldn't be alive when the appointment time finally came around, as all the other oncologists had now decided to give up on me as a lost cause.

Later that same week I was suddenly admitted to a hospital on the Sunshine Coast, as the tumour which was blocking part of my bowel was now causing me extreme pain. The hospital Emergency Department transferred me for a whole-body CT scan, which revealed that the tumour was indeed blocking most of my bowel. This meant that up to this point, even though I was using tubes and enema bags as a toilet mechanism, I now had an obstruction on my bowel itself, which meant that it was virtually impossible for my bowel to operate normally.

The concern at the hospital now at this point was that the pressure from my stomach could rupture my bowel and that would then become a very serious issue.

The hospital team decided that they needed to insert a tube into my nasal passage, which would then be fed down the back of my throat and into my stomach.

This was to form a vacuum suction line, which would be used to try to siphon anything that was in my stomach out, and hope that by doing this, that it might help to release any pressure on my bowel itself.

This was an awful procedure and I really struggled with the tube positioned down inside my throat. I felt like I wanted to choke all the time. I asked the doctor how long this tube would have to remain in place, and I was told that it would have to remain in place until my stomach was completely drained, and the bag, which was now attached to me, no longer filled up with any fluid.

I told the nursing staff that I will monitor the attachment bag myself, and once I see that the tube is no longer siphoning anything from my stomach into the bag, then I would like the tube removed please.

This was around 4.00pm in the afternoon. I lay in my bed, occasionally getting up to go for a walk and still carrying the bag around with me, which was still attached through my nose and down my throat, leading directly into my stomach. It was totally impossible to sleep, and I checked the bag again, at around 4.00am. I could clearly see that since I had last checked the bag at midnight that nothing further had been siphoning into the tube from my stomach, as the measurement level that I had placed on the bag at midnight hadn't changed.

I left the bed to approach the night shift team. I found them all at their hospital transit station, which was located between the various hospital wards. However, at this stage I discovered that they were all asleep on their pillows.

162

I managed to awaken one nurse and I requested if she could please remove the tube from my nose and throat, as it was no longer necessary for it to remain in place, as the drainage from my stomach to the bag was now complete. I was told it will be removed later in the morning.

I replied by telling her "It's fine, I will remove it myself, as I'm in so much discomfort and it's impossible to get any sleep." I was then told to go back to my room, and someone would come and attend to me shortly. I went back to my room and for the next hour I kept continuously pressing the alert button, as I suspected they had all gone back over to sleep once again.

Finally, someone arrived and pulled the tube out of my stomach, up through my throat until it was finally out through my nostrils. I was never so glad to have a tube removed in my entire life. The next morning, I discharged myself from the hospital and I went back to our rental accommodation to try to recover from this awful ordeal.

Now that I knew the full extent of the cancer, I contacted the specialist surgeon again at Albion in Brisbane to see if he could remove four of the deep tumours from inside by back, and close to the large rugby sized football tumour, that was causing me severe discomfort. I explained to him the urgency of the situation, and he agreed to perform the operation to remove the four tumours the following week at the Kawana private hospital.

The agreed costs were eight thousand dollars. This was to cover all the costs associated with the surgeon's fees, the theatre nursing team, the anaesthetist and the hospital fees, including the recovery ward after the anaesthetist and the operation itself.

The following week I went to the hospital as agreed. Prior to going into the theatre for the operation, the surgeon came out to see me before I became fully anaesthetised. He explained the procedure to me, that he was about to carry out, and which I confirmed with him was indeed correct, as it was what we had previously agreed together. I asked him at this stage if it would be possible for him to remove the large tumour which was blocking my anus, however he said he could not carry out that type of procedure as it was a very difficult procedure to perform and from which I might never fully recover from.

I went ahead and I had the four tumours removed in a full day surgery procedure. When the anaesthetic finally started to wear off in the recovery ward the pain was indeed excruciating. I asked the nursing team if I could have some more pain relief and further morphine was administered. My entire back was now covered in pressure pack bandages to try to stop the stitches from busting open and my back from basically, falling apart.

Since so many nerves had been cut whilst the tumours were being removed, even the morphine didn't help me at all, with any type of pain relief or control. After a few hours in the recovery ward, I collected my prescribed pain relief, and I left the hospital. It had certainly been a very long eventful and extremely painful day once again.

Around two weeks later I went back to see the practice nurse at the Caloundra clinic who worked for the surgeon and any of the stitches that hadn't managed to dissolve by themselves in my back, were then each individually removed.

At this stage (even today) my entire back looked like I had just been whipped with a leather strap, from the appearance of the welted scars showing between both of my shoulders.

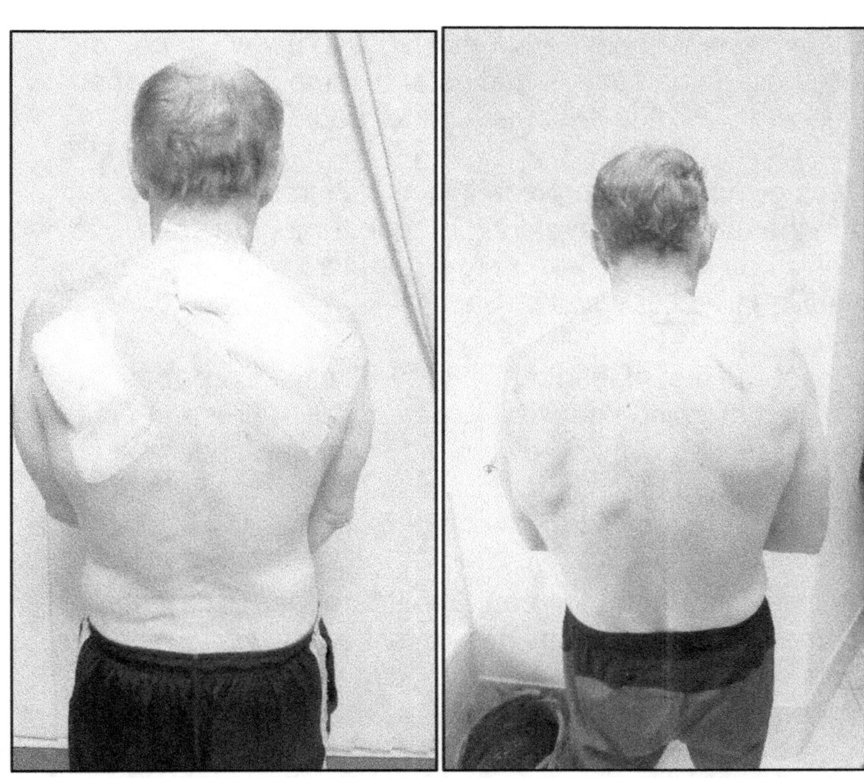

**Pressure Bandages, Scars and Large tumours on
my back in December 2020**

A week later I attended Palliative Care, which is part of the
hospital complex in Caloundra. Currently, I was in such a
bad health condition. The Palliative Care doctor, who met
me, suggested that I should consider remaining in the facility
now, due to the severity of my condition. I reluctantly agreed
to this, and I was then transferred to a private room of the
care facility. I already knew that Palliative Care was where
people were sent for pain relief prior to their passing, and
that it was a way of easing your pain before departure.

This started to cause me some serious concerns.

165

My family went home and returned with my wash bag of toiletries, some spare pyjamas and some car magazines, so at least I would have something to read.

I was given more morphine injections straight into my left arm that now had developed a huge tumour the size of a tennis ball. My son flew up to see me from Melbourne and we all feared the worst.

I spent the first night alone in the Palliative Care room and the next morning I decided to get up out of bed and I put on my dressing gown and blue suede slippers, and I walked around the small courtyard outside, which was also another part of the nearby hospital complex.

As I walked around the courtyard, I stopped for a few moments beside a small tree to rest up, as I was suffering such severe fatigue that I could hardly move. I could no longer sit down anymore either, as the tumour on my bottom was so huge now, and I rested up against the tree using my right arm, as the large tumour on my upper left arm was causing me excruciating pain yet again.

I knew at this point that if I was to remain in this Palliative Care facility much longer, then that is where I would probably die as well. I had previously researched morphine and although I already knew that it assists with temporary pain relief, I also knew that it can cause the cancer to spread around the body. Everything was now pointing towards an end game scenario for me. As I stood leaning up against the tree, I decided to ask the Lord if he could help me to decide on what I should do now, and I would be guided by his advice.

I went back into my room in the Palliative Care ward and both my wife and son arrived soon afterwards to visit me.

I told them I had made my decision, and I wasn't going to remain in Palliative Care, as there was an end game situation arising and I didn't want to pass away in here.

I would rather go home to our rental accommodation.

They fully understood what I was saying, and I told them that I would also tell this to the doctor whenever he or she came around to visit me in the ward later that morning. Not long after they both left the room the doctor came around to carry out the usual morning ward visits to all the inpatients.

Sadly, I could see patients lying in their beds in some of the other rooms who were very seriously ill. I told the doctor that came into my room "Thank you very much for having me here, I really appreciate it, however I don't feel that I want to remain in here any longer, and I'd just prefer to leave now and go home please."

She then told me, "You can't do that, you're not well enough to leave this facility and if you decide to do that, then you won't survive very long outside of Palliative Care without any treatment in your current state." I said "I have already been denied basic hospital treatment, which I have been requesting now for the past three years and which I know can help me to save my own life. If I remain in here, my only option is continuous morphine injections, which will soon kill me quickly anyway, "I'm sorry but I'm grabbing my toiletries and walking out of here now. You're not the Grim Reaper to me." I put all my belongings into a carrier bag, and I walked out of the Care facility. To this day I have never ever heard anything again from Palliative Care, as I suspect they think I have probably passed on by now.

Around this same time, I went to see the brain radiation specialist at the private cancer clinic, who had previously carried out my brain Gamma Knife radiation procedure. At this stage he had already received a copy of my most recent PET scan results from the hospital in Buderim.

He was very shocked that a total of fifteen new brain tumours had developed within only a few months, since I'd had the last brain MRI scan. Sadly, this was the aggressive nature of Metastatic melanoma cancer progression without having any treatment.

He told me that radiation of fifteen tumours at the exact same time was a huge procedure, and that it might have to be completed over two individual procedures, instead of just the one procedure. I told him that whatever you have to do I'm guided as always by your advice, which I totally trust. He asked me what treatment, if any, was I currently on.

I told him that I had not received any hospital treatment whatsoever for the last three years now, as I had been continually refused any further help, from all the oncologists I had approached at two hospitals, both in Brisbane and on the Sunshine Coast.

He then proceeded to ask me if I had ever been on any immunotherapy treatments before. I told him that I was hoping to restart once again on Keytruda immunotherapy next week at a Gold Coast clinic, and I explained to him about the most recent LEAP 004 clinical trial results. I informed him that yes, I had indeed been on Keytruda immunotherapy previously, at the same time as he had completed my first Gamma Knife radiation procedure in March 2017.

I told him that I had been taken off the treatment, as the oncologist at that time said that it was no longer working for me, as a new tumour had appeared, and I wasn't so sure that this was indeed correct.

I continued to tell him that I had been trying nonstop for the past three years, to get back onto either Keytruda or Opdivo immunotherapy treatment again, but that I'd had no success whatsoever finding any help anywhere from any oncologists at any hospitals.

This was even after I had provided them with solid proof, showing that either treatment would work for me from the results I had confirmed, of the genetic testing I had carried out at both laboratories in Germany and in the USA.

He then looked at me and said, "So they took you off the immunotherapy treatment?" I replied "Yes, that's correct." He then asked me if I had been prescribed any steroids at the same time, that I was on the immunotherapy treatment. I said "Yes, I was prescribed Dexamethasone for several months." He turned around at his desk and looked at me with a shocked appearance on his face.

He then said "No" I replied "Yes, I was prescribed a course of Dexamethasone for several months and it had caused me severe insomnia and I had been unable to sleep properly because of its effects." He turned around once again with a shocked look on his face and said, "The immunotherapy treatment that you were receiving at that same time would never have worked for you, because Dexamethasone is a steroid that stops the immunotherapy from actually working its magic." I could not believe what I was hearing. I asked," Was that really possible?" He said, "It could never have worked for you, it would be impossible and I'm so sorry that this has happened to you."

He said that he had instructed the treating oncologist at that time, after the brain radiation procedure had been completed, to prescribe me the Dexamethasone for seven days only then cease. It's function is to be taken for seven days only, to deal with the swelling inside your brain that occurs after the severe radiation treatment.

I was totally astounded at this latest shock news.

After I received my hospital medical history, I later discovered a copy of the original letter that he had written to the oncologist after the brain radiation procedure was completed and it did state, "For Dexamethasone 4mg daily for 7 days then cease."

Treatment: Gamma Knife Radiosurgery 7/3/17

This is a treatment summary for your records.

Today Robin has received Gamma Knife to 7 brain metastases. Although he remains clinically stable, there was significant progression since his previous MRI only a few weeks before.

Today the left temporal, right posterior frontal and left parietal lesions were larger and new smaller lesions in the left parietal, left putamen, right cerebellum, and right posterior frontal lobes were seen. All lesions were treated with each receiving 18-20Gy.

Robin tolerated treatment well but of course was upset by these findings. For dexamethasone 4mg daily for 7 days and then cease. I have arranged to see him again in 2 months with a repeat MRI brain. I have recommended that he does not drive until my next review.

The Radiologist instructions to the Oncologist Dexamethasone for 7 days then cease

He then told me that he would arrange for me to have another Gamma Knife brain radiation procedure, as soon as possible, due to the fact if I was simply placed onto a hospital queue it might take several months, before I would receive the treatment that I desperately needed.

He feared that if we didn't act fast, then sadly it would be too late to do anything at all to help save me. Within a few days he contacted me again to advise me that the Gamma Knife brain radiation had now been arranged for December 23rd, which was two days before Christmas. I thanked him very much for arranging this so quickly for me and I confirmed that I would indeed be attending on that day.

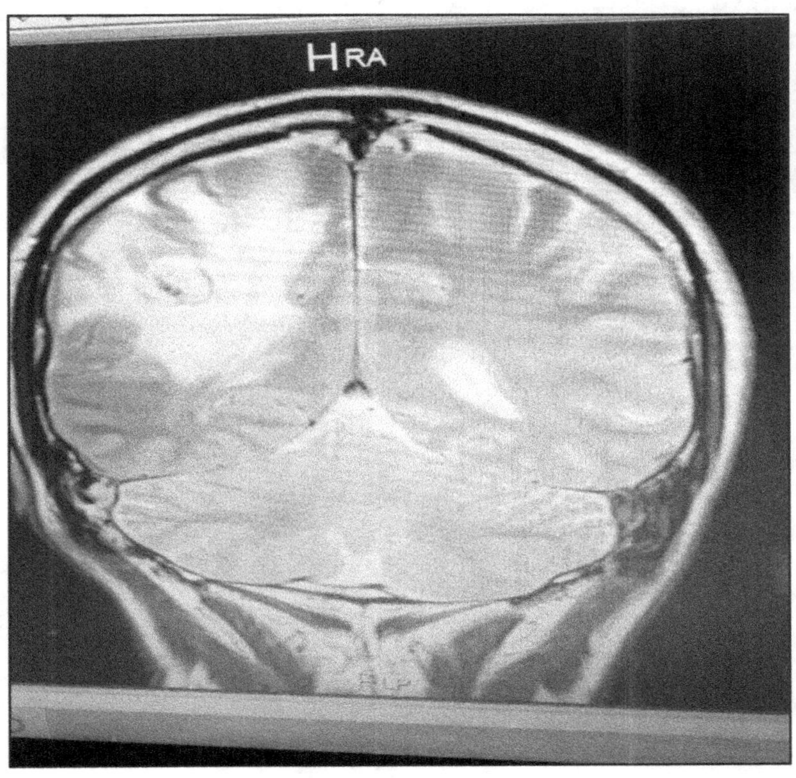

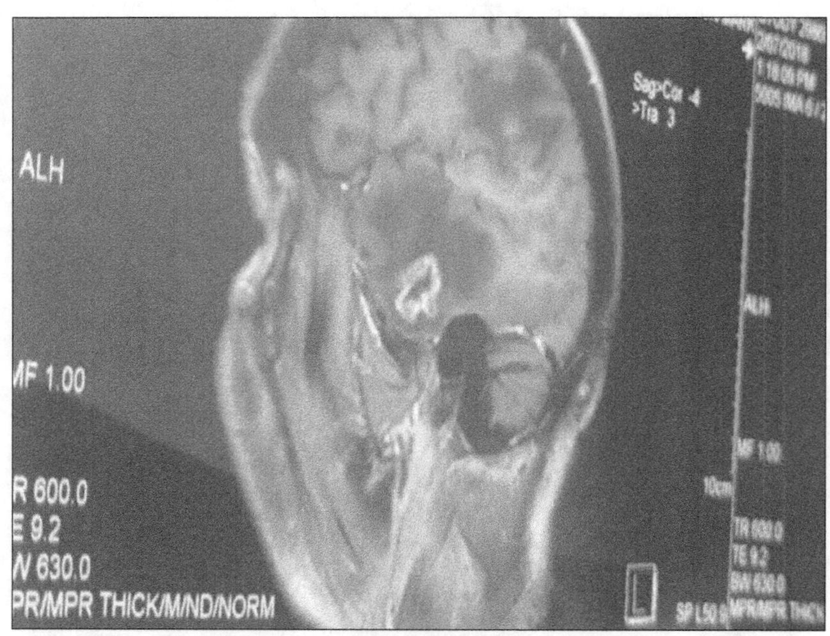

Brain Tumour MRI Scan images

ANOTHER RAY OF HOPE

At this point I hadn't met the other oncologist yet on the Gold Coast, as we had only been communicating to each other via email. I had also asked him if it would be possible to have the V-Tec trial drug injected into each of my tumours individually. This is a type of remodelled herpes virus that had been going through clinical trials. The virus was injected into the centre of each tumour, in an attempt, to destroy them. I had been researching it and I also discovered that some of these trials were being conducted at the Peter Mac Cancer Centre in Melbourne. I decided to contact the Peter Mac directly, to see if it might be possible to have this treatment carried out there and I could then stay with my son, who lives in Melbourne for the duration of the procedures.

Unfortunately, they replied, that up to this stage they were only having very limited success with the new drug, and due to the very large number of tumours, that I now had in my body, it would be impossible to inject into every one of them, and they said "Sorry, but we won't be able to help you now."

The Gold Coast oncologist said that it would be best if we discussed all this at our meeting, which had now been arranged for later that same week. During the past few weeks, I had continued to email the Federal Health minister in Canberra daily, begging him for help that I could be given the treatment that I knew might just help me to extend my life. Unfortunately, as always, I could never receive any response. I was so disappointed that everything I was trying was being totally ignored. It was heart-breaking.

In my correspondence to the Federal Health Minister, I told him that, we as a country can donate millions of dollars each year to other countries, but we can't provide basic treatment to our own people who need it the most. It was an absolute disgrace to be treating citizens of our country in this manner.

I contacted my two sisters and my cousin in Northern Ireland, as they were already aware of the severity of my health condition at this time. They also started to take up my case for me and they started writing personally to the health minister and to the oncologist at the local hospital on the Sunshine Coast in Queensland who had pretty much sentenced me to death.

Sadly, there was no response from the Federal Health Minister, which was now to be expected, and the hospital oncologist simply replied stating that everything that could possibly be done for me had already been done, and because I had already failed several treatments (which I later proved to them was completely wrong) including Opdivo and Keytruda, which were both immunotherapy treatments, it would be totally impossible for anything to work for me now.

My family decided to continue to step up their campaign to try to get me help. They approached a local councillor, who was a close friend of the family. He knew Lord Empey in the House of Lords in London, and he contacted Lord Empey directly, to ask if he could possibly take up my case, to request help to try to keep me alive. Lord Empey took up my case and he wrote personally to the Australian Federal Health Minister from the House of Lords at Westminster, requesting that I may be considered for treatment, as I was in a very bad way at this time, with having no access to treatment for the last three years.

He told him that both, my family and I were well respected people in Northern Ireland, from the constituency that he was very proud to represent.

Lord Empey of Shandon Kt. OBE.

I have been contacted by friends and relatives of Mr Robin Smyth who are very concerned about his very serious illness and his inability, so far, to receive the treatment he believes can prolong his life. Mr Smyth originally came from County Down in Northern Ireland, which I am proud to represent.

I am attaching some of the details of his long battle with illness, but it all boils down to whether or not he can access Opdivo.

It is believed that this drug Can shrink his tumour and thereby prolong life.

Having served as a Minister myself, I know only too well that resources are not unlimited, and in the case of health, one is always listening to medical advice. That said, this case is at a critical point and your intervention in this matter would be greatly appreciated by all the Smyth family.

I do hope you can help Robin and his family.

Kind regards

Whilst this campaign was underway, I had now travelled to meet with the oncologist on the Gold Coast, to discuss my referral to him from the Australian Melanoma Institute in Sydney and the LEAP004 clinical trial. He was already very aware of this trial, as he was currently treating several other Queensland patients with the exact same immunotherapy treatment. We discussed my most recent whole body PET scan, and he knew the severity of just how serious my cancer condition now was.

175

I discussed the T-Vec virus injections, and I asked if he could help me with this, even as a trial as I had nothing left to lose at this point. He too was of the same opinion as the Peter Mac Cancer centre, that due to the multiple tumours that were now present in my body that even if the virus was supplied compassionately, it would be impossible to inject it into each tumour individually, without causing my death and he wasn't prepared to do this, which I understood and respected.

I was hoping we could have at least tried six tumours, as the ones on my arm, anus and on my back were horrific at this stage and I wasn't able to have any sleep, and as a result of the sleep deprivation, I was now suffering from extreme exhaustion. I was almost unable to walk very far without some form of support.

I had even considered trying to obtain medicinal cannabis to try to help ease my pain, and to possibly get some sleep, but I didn't proceed with this as my research showed that it interfered with the immunotherapy treatment, and it would make it less effective at reprogramming the immune system, to find and eradicate the cancer cells.

At this stage I didn't want to do or use anything that might stop the treatment from working for me.

We discussed the Opdivo immunotherapy treatment which I had been continually refused by all the other hospitals. He was very aware that both the Opdivo and the Keytruda were very similar drugs, with the only real difference being that they were manufactured by two different pharmaceutical companies.

I asked him if he could possibly obtain the Opdivo immunotherapy compassionately for me from the company who supplied the treatment, but he said that this would be impossible. We discussed the Yervoy, or 'Ippy', as it is also referred to as, and I said that this particular drug had almost killed me in 2017 and I would never take it again, as I would not be confident that I would be able to survive it a second time around.

He was already aware of the severity of this drug, as he had several other patients who had also experienced similar side effects to what I had just gone through. I told him about the Smecta medication that I had researched and used to treat my colitis and how I had cured it myself, and unlike the previous oncologists that I had discussed it with, he was genuinely interested, and took notes of what I was discussing with him. I was pleased that my information might just save another person's life, at some stage in the future.

We then discussed the other treatment called Lenvatinib, which was the second drug that had been used in the LEAP 004 clinical trial, along with the Keytruda immunotherapy. The idea behind the immunotherapy treatment is that it attempts to reprogram the body's own immune system into recognising and then destroying the pathogens, which are the cancer cells inside the body and then the Lymphocytes, which make up the "fighting soldiers" of the body's T-Cells, then attack and eliminate them.

My immune system had already been totally depleted from the unnecessary chemotherapy I was given in 2010. The chemotherapy not only tries to eliminate the cancer cells, but it also destroys every normal cell in the body at the very same time. What is not told to patients is that this chemical poisoning does not remove the cancer stem cells.

What this means is that although it might kill some of the actual cancer cells, it does not destroy the cancer stem cells, and because of this the cancer can return a second time around, and this is the reason why, in a lot of cases people sadly get their cancers returning viciously once again.

It's very similar to trying to remove a weed from your garden. You try to pull out the weed and only the leaves come away, leaving the root still in the ground. This means that the weed will regrow again, because the root itself is still there. This is the exact same with cancer. When the cancer stem cells remain in the body, then at some stage the cancer will start to regrow once more, but usually more aggressively the second time around.

The other treatment, Lenvatinib is designed to cut off the feed supply to the tumour, in an attempt, to starve it to death. The cancer tumour grows, because it feeds itself off the body's own blood supply. This is very similar to an octopus, which feeds itself through using its tentacles.

The tumour puts out feeler roots and reaches into the body's own blood supply, to continue to feed itself. The Lenvatinib is designed to cut off this feed supply through the tentacles, and in so doing starves the cancer tumour to death and destroys it.

I told the oncologist I wasn't sure how long I would be able to afford the treatment, as we had already sold our home and sadly, we were now only barely able to afford to pay our rent each week.

I knew that paying for the treatment was only one expense as the oncologist also had to be paid for his consultation, hospital fees, nursing staff and other related costs.

This would then add a further six hundred dollars to each infusion. He then told me that the cost of the treatment would be six thousand five hundred dollars every three weeks and the Lenvatinib would be an additional four thousand dollars on top of this. This amounted to approximately ten thousand six hundred dollars every three weeks, plus a four hour round travel trip to the Gold Coast, not including the fuel costs.

Shortly after this, he commenced to tell me something that no other oncologist had ever revealed to me at any stage before, and which left me shocked, angry and extremely dismayed. He asked me if I was aware of what a 'capped' Pharmaceutical scheme was. I replied that no, I hadn't heard of this type of scheme, and could he please explain to me in more detail what this was? He continued to tell me that the Keytruda, which was the immunotherapy treatment I had already researched in 2017 and which I had requested to be given, then sadly only to be taken off it again a few months later after I was told that it wasn't working for me, or the Opdivo treatment, could both be accessed through this scheme, from each of the two respective pharmaceutical companies.

The treatment was supplied at a total 'capped' amount of sixty thousand dollars. What this meant was that, as an enrolled patient with the respective pharmaceutical company, once a patient had reached paying this 'capped' threshold of sixty thousand dollars, then the remainder of the treatment (if you were responding to the treatment at the time) would then be provided to you totally free of charge ongoing.

I couldn't believe what I was now hearing.

I asked the oncologist, was I correct in my understanding that what he had just told me was, that the most I would pay for my treatment in total ongoing would be sixty thousand dollars. He replied "Yes, that is correct, the maximum you will pay will be sixty thousand dollars for either of the two immunotherapy treatments that you decide to use, however you will still be required to pay the additional associated fees for my consultation, the clinic itself, my staff and all the medical items that are necessary to provide you with the treatment."

I said, "I am totally flabbergasted to hear this information." He then asked me, "Why would that be." I replied, "For the last three years I have been continually told by all the other oncologists that I have attended, that the cost of either of these two treatments would be in excess of two hundred thousand dollars each year and I knew that I could never afford to fund this, as I had already spent over five hundred thousand dollars on various treatments worldwide, trying to keep myself alive."

I said, "In all these years I have lost everything, including my home, my savings, my superannuation, the cars that I all hand built from scratch to enjoy should I reach retirement, and now I am totally penniless as a result."

I said "That's a total disgrace, not only did I develop this horrific cancer in the first place from being prescribed unnecessary chemotherapy, that destroyed me, but then afterwards trying to keep myself alive with little or no support, no compensation, no apology, it's been a shocking road to have been on and I'm still on this same road today."

I told him that I was very much appreciative, to be told this news and I would like to proceed with commencing the immunotherapy treatment immediately, as it was my last hope.

I said that if I had known this information in 2017, when I was taken off the Keytruda, I would have commenced this scheme back then, and I might have recovered from this horrible disease and still also owned my home and possibly had some savings left as well.

I knew at this time I could only just manage to afford this treatment if I could pay it off each treatment day, until I had reached the agreed 'capped' amount. He replied that yes, this was indeed possible. I told him that I would be able to afford the Keytruda but unfortunately, I would not be able to afford the extra Lenvatinib medication, even though it was also going to be 'capped' at thirty thousand dollars. Both treatments would then have cost me a total of ninety thousand dollars, which I knew I would not be able to afford to pay plus the additional clinic fees.

I asked if I could commence this treatment as soon as possible, as I was so ill at this stage. He told me that the treatment would have to be ordered into the clinic pharmacy first, from the pharmaceutical company, and that it could be delivered to them the following week. I said this would be very much appreciated and the agreed treatment scheme would then be to have regular infusions every three weeks, with mandatory blood tests in advance and an oncologist appointment before each treatment.

Each treatment and the associated costs would require to be paid at the commencement of each procedure, which I also fully understood.

It was now early December 2020 and I travelled to the Gold Coast clinic where I met the oncologist once again for a consultation update, after which I was then introduced to the various nursing staff.

I was also shown the location of the clinic pharmacy where the payments would need to be completed, prior to having infusions carried out, and then I proceeded to receive my first treatment of Keytruda since I was taken off it in 2017. I had a sincere feeling of relief as soon as I had this initial treatment completed once again.

In the following few days, I decided that I would commence further research on the other medication known as Lenvatinib, as it had also been the other medication on the LEAP 004 clinical trial. I discovered that this treatment was available for purchase from overseas and the cost of the medication was approximately ten thousand dollars per year. I decided that I would place an order for it straight away as I wasn't able to afford the thirty thousand dollars which was being charged for the same treatment here in Australia.

I obtained a prescription, which would then enable it to be imported through the Australian Customs, and I promptly ordered the medication, which was delivered very swiftly ten days later.

This meant that I was now able to commence this daily treatment immediately after receiving it. I had already checked out the supplier, and the company was listed on the New York Stock Exchange.

After this, I was satisfied at this point that it was being manufactured by a reputable pharmaceutical company and not just another online scamming fraud. In addition to this I had found another product known as IP6. This herb was an antioxidant that had shown success in helping to treat and prevent cancer by slowing down the production of the actual cancer cells themselves. It had also shown an ability to bind to certain minerals, which decreased the risk of colon cancer. I found a very reputable supplier of this IP6 and I ordered several months' supply and I commenced taking this supplement each day. I have continued to take this supplement daily since then.

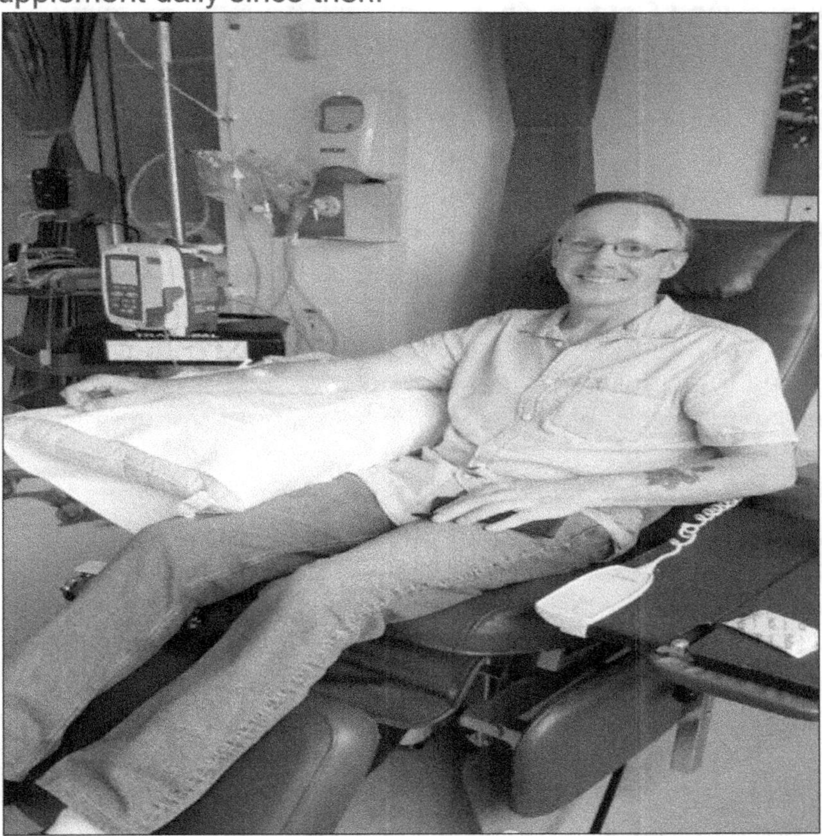

Robin starting Keytruda Immunotherapy again privately on the Gold Coast in December 2020

EVIDENCE I WAS CORRECT ONCE AGAIN

With Christmas rapidly approaching, the date had been set for my second brain radiation treatment at the hospital in Brisbane. It was arranged for December the 23rd. I left the Sunshine Coast at 4.30am, as the procedure had been booked for a 6.00am arrival time. I arrived at the Queensland Gamma Knife Centre in Brisbane ten minutes early and I waited outside the entrance to the building.

There were several other patients waiting on the same bench with me, and we chatted about the procedures that we were all going to be having carried out during the day. Quite a few patients were going to be having this procedure for the very first time, and I tried to share my previous experience with them, in the hope that it might just help to relief some of the anxiety they were all clearly suffering. I shared the swelling issues and how the Dexamethasone drug would probably cause them to have insomnia, as it was a drug that was sometimes used by young students trying to keep themselves awake, whilst studying for their school examinations. I also chatted about my use of the Frankincense extract Boswellia Serrata, and how I found that it had helped me during my own recovery.

I was extremely nervous myself, as this was now going to be my second time around and I was even more concerned this time than I had been previously, as I now had fifteen brain tumours inside my skull, that were all going to be struck one by one, hopefully with pinpoint accuracy, by a radiation laser machine.

I was worried that by 'blowing up' fifteen tumours at once inside my brain, that it might leave me permanently brain damaged or even death could occur, as a result of such a high amount of radiation being delivered to my brain at the same time.

When the main doors opened at 6.00 am, we all entered the building together, wishing each other the very best of luck for each of our respective procedures. After I had changed into my hospital gown, I was then instructed to make my way to the Medical Imaging department of the hospital, for yet another brain scan. I was told that the radiologist, who would be carrying out my procedure later that morning needed updated imaging, to ensure precision accuracy, in order for each tumour to be targeted successfully. After this scan was finished, I was then transferred to the fit-out room. This is where the metal frame is screwed into your skull to secure it to your head. This is the most painful part of the procedure, as the frame once again, is fitted directly into your skull with four steel screws, which are inserted with a battery-operated drill, fitted with a Phillips Head screwdriver attachment bit.

Once this frame was secured into place, I was transferred to another hospital bed where the frame on my skull was then clamped to the steel framework of the bed itself. This meant I couldn't move my head even half a millimetre. My arms were also secured to the side of the frame and then the whole trolley frame is pushed inside the radiation machine. I just hoped that this time I didn't have a fly land on my nose which had happened to me on the last Gamma Knife experience.

I prayed again that the good Lord would help me to survive what was about to happen to me.

I asked that the necessary skills would be given to the Radiation specialist, and that he would be successful with his procedures on my brain.

After several hours inside the radiation machine, I heard the voice talking to me through the inbuilt speakers, telling me that it was all over now. I had done very well again and that I would be brought out of the machine very soon and the frame would be removed from my skull.

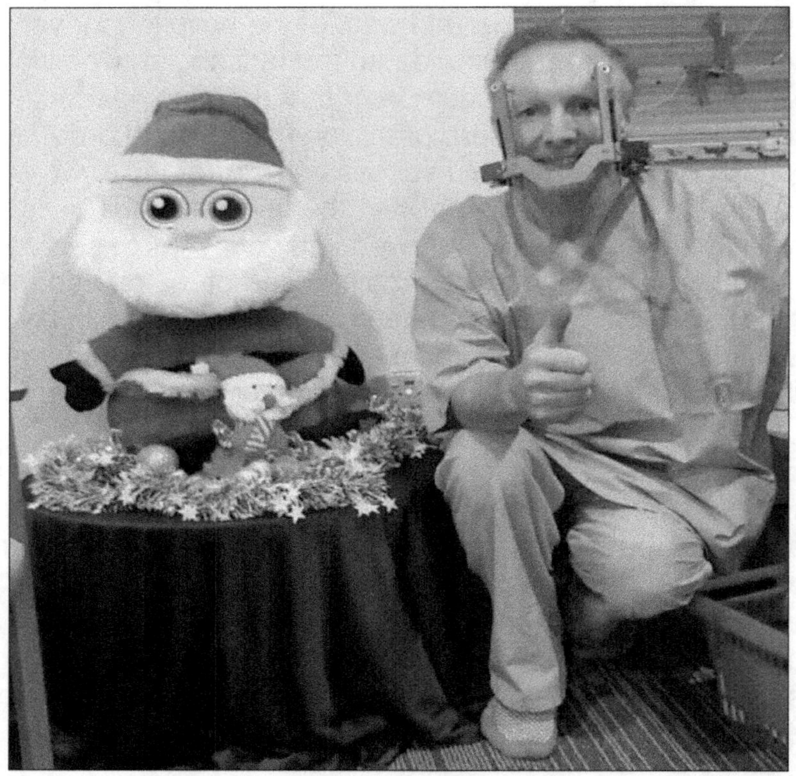

The Steel Frame screwed directly into my Skull for the Radiation on 15 Brain Tumours

I had managed once again to survive another serious onslaught and I was very thankful for it.

The battery powered drill was produced once again and the metal frame was unscrewed from my skull, in the four places where it had been secured earlier.

I was thankful once again to the good Lord for guiding the specialists and helping me to survive yet another procedure on the fifteen new brain tumours.

I then changed back again from my theatre gown into my normal dress clothing, before I left the hospital to return home to our rental accommodation on the Sunshine Coast. My head at this time felt like it had just gone through fifteen rounds of being beaten by a world heavyweight boxing champion or a travelling boxing tent troupe.

The next day being Christmas Eve my wife took me to a beachside town called Scarborough, where I spent the next few days recuperating from what I had just gone through.

This time the aftermath was even more severe, given the fact that previously I had been dealing with seven brain tumours, and this time I had managed to survive fifteen brain tumours, all being struck at the same time. I was so weak that I was struggling to even try to walk. I couldn't even put my own shoes on, and I relied on shuffling my feet along in a pair of blue suede slippers. I was totally unable to lift my legs to walk in a normal manner.

The next morning was Christmas day and I got up early at first sunrise. I put on my slippers and left the complex to shuffle my way to the edge of the nearby beach.

As I sat on the park bench, I pondered over what I had just gone through once again.

I hoped that the new treatment I had just started would help me to survive, and to preserve my life a little bit longer.

After a few days away we travelled back home again, only to discover that the house that we were currently renting at this time, was to be re-occupied by its owners, as it was their rental investment property.

We had been told initially that we could have our lease for six months, and if needed, we could extend it again for yet another six months.

Sadly, this was not to be the case, and we now had the extra stress of trying to find another place to live, in the midst, of all this turmoil, as I was still extremely weak, to even try to begin moving our furniture and personal belongings around once more.

I contacted a close friend of mine, who knew some people who were involved with real estate rental properties, and he spoke with them on my behalf, and within two weeks of our four-week deadline to vacate, we had managed to find another rental property, which wasn't too far from where we were currently staying at Kawana. It was ironic that I was born on the 19th at number nineteen, and both the consecutive rental properties where we had stayed at, were also both number nineteen as well.

At this time, I was still taking my daily Boswellia Serrata Frankincense extract capsules as I didn't use the Dexamethasone medication again, from the knowledge that I had now learnt earlier about its anti-immunotherapy effects.

I didn't want anything at this point, to interfere with the treatment that I had just commenced a week earlier on the Gold Coast.

On the 30th of December 2020 I once again travelled to the Gold Coast Cancer centre to have my second Keytruda treatment, and thirteen thousand dollars paid to date.

I decided to start investigating if this treatment could possibly be provided to me at another cancer facility on the Sunshine Coast, which would be much closer, instead of the five hours travel that I required at this time, through heavy city traffic to the Gold Coast treatment centre, for each infusion.

After a brief search I found a private facility located at Buderim on the Sunshine Coast, which was less than a twenty-minute drive from my rental accommodation.

I contacted the facility to arrange an appointment with one of their oncologists, who specialised in treating melanoma cancers. I was offered an appointment at this clinic, and the cost of the initial consultation with the oncologist was quoted at five hundred dollars.

A week later I travelled to the Buderim clinic, and I attended my first appointment with this oncologist. Prior to this meeting, I had already looked up the reviews left by his other patients, and I was satisfied with what I had been reading from them. I shared with him my medical history from the unnecessary chemotherapy poisoning in 2011, up to my present situation, trying to fight off this terrible disease.

I asked if it might be possible for me to continue my current immunotherapy treatment at the Buderim clinic.

I also asked if he might be able to obtain the treatment from the pharmaceutical company on compassionate grounds.

Sadly, once again this wasn't to be the case. He informed me that the Keytruda treatment plan I was currently on with the pharmaceutical company, could still be continued at the Buderim clinic.

After further discussions, we agreed that the consultancy costs, nursing staff and the medical materials required to provide me with the treatment, would be the same as I was already paying to have the treatment administered at the Gold Coast clinic.

When the next scheduled three-week treatment time came around once again, I travelled back to the Gold Coast clinic.

I discussed with the oncologist about my plans to switch my treatment facilities to the Buderim clinic and I thanked him and his team for all their help to me. The treating oncologist had no issues with this changeover and wished me well.

The time had also come around again for our rental accommodation switch, and with the help of some friends we managed to move everything that we owned to the neighbouring suburb of Kawana. This was to become our temporary home once again for another six months.

At this time, I could clearly see that the treatment I had chosen as my therapy was already starting to work its magic on me. Some of the very large tumours that I had on my back, which were the ones that no surgeon would even attempt to remove before, were very visibly starting to shrink. I had already decided to take some photographs of these tumours on my back, before commencing the new immunotherapy treatment.

There were now very noticeable differences between them, when comparing both sets of photographs.

Over the years I had also learnt from reading my own blood test reports, how to monitor my body's lactate LDH levels. I had found that higher levels of LDH were an obvious sign of a renewed increase in the cancer cell activity in the body.

When I had my blood tests completed at the beginning of my treatment, the LDH level was showing a reading of 362. The latest blood test reports were now showing that the levels had dramatically reduced to only 204.

This was a very significant drop, in a very short period, which indicated to me that the treatment was working as I had already expected it would.

I was still not having any success from either of the local politicians that I had been regularly emailing. I sent further emails again to the Federal Health Minister with no response.

I emailed the Queensland State Health Minister every single day in January 2021 and never once in over thirty emails, did I ever receive any reply, other than an automated response, telling me that my correspondence had been received.

Lord Empey from the House of Lords at Westminster once again contacted the Australian Federal Health Minister regarding my current health situation.

I later discovered that in fact the Federal Health Minister had indeed forwarded the matter on to the Queensland Premier who had then forwarded it on to the State Health Minister who in turn had then sent it to the Head of the Queensland Health department for the Brisbane area.

191

Finally, I managed to eventually receive a response from the regional Health director informing me again that everything that could be done for me had already been done and that regrettably nothing else could be offered to me by way of any future treatments. It was now the end of January 2021. I responded to this reply by return email. It was now time for me to once again provide proof showing how this treatment was already working for me, which it would have been doing all along, if I had not been wrongly taken of it in 2017. I didn't need any medical scans or imaging to prove this. The photographs themselves, or as a picture speaks a thousand words, very clearly showed my tumours both before commencing the Keytruda immunotherapy treatment, and then the same tumours four weeks later. The changes showed a significant difference in appearance. The large rugby sized tumour, and the other massive tumour at the top of my back under my left shoulder, which was in the scapular region, had shrunk in size by almost fifty per cent.

I had now made the arranged transfer from the Gold Coast cancer clinic to the Buderim cancer clinic. I was attending this clinic now, every three weeks, which was the standard immunotherapy treatment programme and I had also started to put some weight back onto my body again, which was helping me to rebuild myself, and I was finally starting to feel stronger again as well and most definitely not as tired I had been for so long previously. I also requested from the administrator at the clinic, all my treatment information in relation to the agreed 'capped' amount. This showed what I had already paid to date for the treatments I had received at the Gold Coast clinic, and the amount still owing from the sixty thousand dollars 'capped' amount. This was the total amount that I had agreed to, before the treatment would be supplied to me free of charge. I also received my patient pharmaceutical ID number, which was used by the cancer clinic as their reference, for them to receive my regular pharmaceutical supply.

NEVER GIVE UP

I was not simply going to just let this matter of being denied basic public health treatment disappear. I had paid my taxes for many years as a working citizen, and I was entitled to be treated like any other citizen. Sadly, this was now being denied to me and from March 2017 it felt like I was being treated as a second-class citizen by the health department.

The very first treatment that I had selected and requested for myself at that time, which was the immunotherapy Keytruda, I had now shown everyone, that it had indeed been the correct choice for me. I should never have been taken off it in 2017 when an oncologist told me that it wasn't working for me. This was so wrong and yet another complete medical blunder which cost me in excess of five hundred thousand dollars, trying to keep myself alive in any way I possibly could. I had lost my business, my home, my savings, my superannuation, the cars that I had built and the numerous operations that have left me permanently scarred for life, including the loss of my salivary gland, from yet another horrific and unnecessary medical failure.

Sadly, my only income left now was a small fortnightly disability pension which I am still trying to survive on to this day. I decided to continue pursuing for some form of justice, as it was now impossible to keep funding the six thousand dollars every three weeks for the Keytruda infusions alone.

I contacted a good friend of mine, who was also a Justice of the Peace to request his help, as I was going to try and arrange a mediation meeting in Brisbane.

This was going to be a meeting between myself and the oncologists from the hospital, including the oncologist who had given me the chemical poisoning in the very first instance, the one who had triggered this whole situation. As far as I was concerned, the treatment which I had originally chosen for myself in March 2017, and which I had been taken off only a few months later, had very clearly resulted in this whole saga continuing. I now had the proof that this was clearly the correct treatment for me for me all along and I should not be denied it any longer. I had already shown the evidence from my own photographs, which I had taken both before commencing the treatment in December and then again in January with undeniable evidence of success. No scans were even necessary at this stage. The images themselves were very clearly enough evidence on their own behalf.

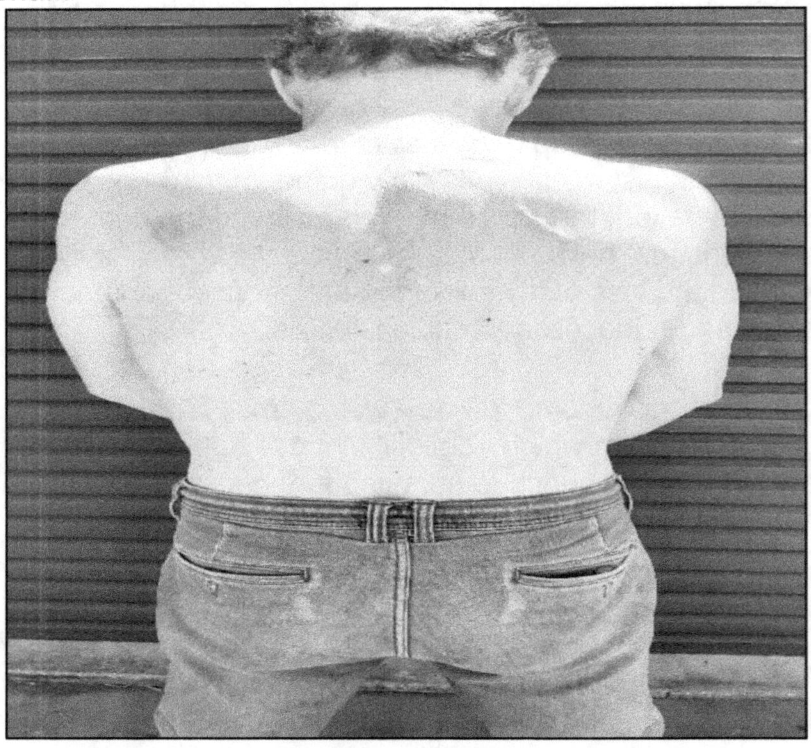

Proof that the Tumours were all shrinking

194

On the 26th of February 2021 I received another email communication from the health department which suggested that, yes, I should indeed meet with the oncologists in Brisbane to discuss this situation further. I replied by telling them that I would only agree to attend a meeting on the condition that I was placed back onto the original immunotherapy treatment again, that I had been taken off in 2017 as I now had supplied them with enough photographic evidence that the treatment was indeed working for me and that the images which I had supplied in the last communication certainly provided enough evidence that this was indeed correct.

A mediation meeting was arranged by the health department for the 29th of March 2021, at which both oncologists, my Justice of the Peace friend, and other witnesses would attend. I once again replied stating that I would only agree to an attendance at the meeting if the immunotherapy treatment was going to be provided to me again.

One week later I received another reply from a clinical nursing consultant from the hospital in Brisbane informing me that if I attended the hospital the following week and met with the oncologist, that I would indeed be commencing my original treatment once again, that very same day. Finally, I was getting somewhere with all my persistence, and the support and help of others along this journey.

I contacted everyone concerned and informed them that the planned mediation meeting at the hospital in Brisbane between all the prearranged parties was no longer necessary, as an agreement had now been reached and the scheduled meeting had been cancelled.

After having already paid for five cycles of Keytruda immunotherapy, which amounted to thirty-two thousand, five hundred dollars. I contacted the cancer clinic at Buderim, to advise them of the most recent updates, and I also requested from them that I might be able to receive a confirmation of the total amount, that I had already paid to date for my treatment. I also wanted confirmation, that should I ever be taken off this treatment again at any hospital for any reason, then the amount that I had already paid would be credited from the agreed 'capped' amount of sixty thousand dollars.

In March 2021 I travelled back again to Brisbane to attend this scheduled hospital meeting. Once again, I walked along the now very familiar corridor to the cancer department. This was a walk I hadn't been on now for several years, and it was nice to see that there was still a nice selection of beautiful paintings adorning the corridor walls.

I had already completed the mandatory blood tests a few days earlier, which were required before any immunotherapy treatment was administered, and I knew that everything was fine to go ahead with the planned treatment.

I approached the reception desk to advise them of my arrival, and to await my prearranged appointment with the oncologist, whom I hadn't seen now for several years. The young lady receptionist at the desk asked me "Which doctor"? I replied "Yes, that's me the Witch Doctor" which was a reference to what some people had been calling me recently, as they couldn't understand how I was still able to be alive. She answered, "Which doctor are you here to see"? I joked back to the girl, "Oh yes sorry I'm here to see Dr. X, I have an appointment." The young girl smiled and told me to please take a seat, and she would let the Doctor know that I had arrived for my appointment.

Whilst I was waiting for my appointment with the oncologist, I recognised one of the nursing team in the distance. I gave her a wave and she came hurriedly towards me and gave me a huge hug. It was a very emotional reunion, because the last time she had seen me at the hospital a few years earlier I was in a very bad way lying on a hospital bed, and nobody had expected that they would ever see me again. She was ecstatic to see me, and it turned out that she was the nurse who would also be administering my treatment again that very same day. It really was a fantastic feeling and she joked by asking me "Have your dad jokes improved?" She told me that she had been reading her schedule of patients for the day and she had recognised my name on her list, and that's why she had been watching out for me in the waiting area of the Cancer Department. It was a nice reunion once again.

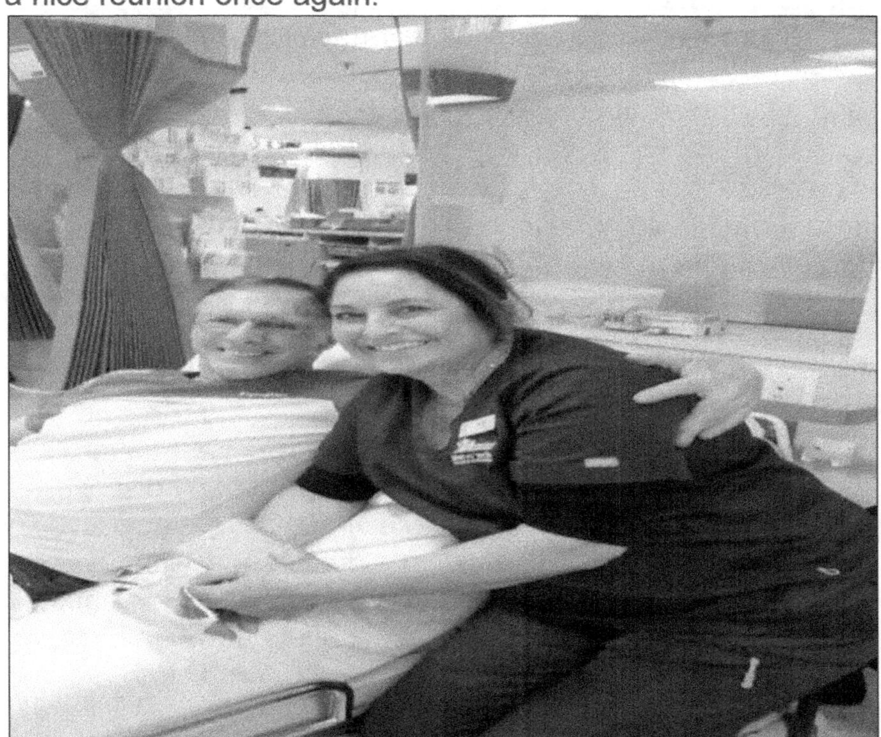

Robin reunited again with Trish at the Hospital

Shortly after this I was called into the oncologist's office. It was a nervous time for everyone since over the last few years everybody had been expecting me to pass on, and for me to be able to make an appearance again in this office was quite simply amazing, that I had made it this far.

The oncologist then commenced to tell me "You now qualify to be given the Keytruda treatment once again, as it appears that you now meet the PBS criteria, as you seem to be responding well to the treatment, judging by the recent reports that I have been looking at. You definitely are a miracle man, as I haven't known anyone with this particular terminal illness survive as long as you have." I said "Yes, the treatment which I had originally selected for myself in 2017 is working very well once again. I just wish that you hadn't prescribed me with that Dexamethasone steroid for so long at that time, otherwise I might never have been taken off this treatment in the first place and suffered so much devastation and heartbreak afterwards."

The oncologist said, "Well we beg to differ on that, as I didn't prescribe it to you that long." I replied, "I'm sorry, but you did." We both moved on from this and I signed the necessary paperwork that was required, in order for me to begin the treatment once again. I asked if my blood results were okay. It was confirmed that they were fine.

I then asked if it would be possible for me to be transferred onto a six-week treatment cycle, as I had already discovered that some patients, who were receiving this treatment every three weeks, were now receiving a double treatment every six weeks and there appeared to be no obvious side effects from doing this. It would also make it a lot easier when trying to insert the cannula needles into my war-torn veins.

It was becoming more and more difficult now and most times I attended to have treatment, the staff suggested that should really consider having a Porta Cath fitted into my chest, which I didn't want, due to the regular maintenance that was required with it.

The oncologist agreed to this and told me that I could commence the six weekly cycles from that day forward. I left the office, and I made my way around to the nearby treatment room and there I had my first infusion of Keytruda since July 2017, which was almost four years earlier. I spent the next few hours having my infusion, and chatting again with my nurse friend Trish, as we obviously had so much to catch up on, as it had been so long since I had last been there and the circumstances surrounding it.

A new CT scan was arranged by the oncologist for the 3rd of June 2021. This was to reassess the latest situation regarding my cancer tumours, considering that only eight months earlier in October 2020, prior to commencing my immunotherapy I had approximately ninety tumours throughout my entire body, stretching from my head right down to my calves.

The report from the latest whole body CT scan concluded that there had been multiple reductions in my tumours, both in the size and also, in the number. Some tumours had reduced in size from originally being twenty-seven millimetres down now to only eight millimetres and those that were showing up on the previous PET scan, as large as thirty millimetres, were now down to only twelve millimetres.

The massive tumours that I had originally on my thigh, chest, left arm, anus and including the rugby ball sized one on my back had all virtually disappeared.

199

There were no new brain tumours showing up anywhere, and the remaining two brain tumours that were displaying on the scans were regarded as being stable in their appearance, and quite possibly only scar tissue, that had been left over from previous tumours that had already been destroyed during the Gamma Knife radiation procedure.

For me, to see this result was an incredible response. It once again confirmed that the decision not to give in to the beast had been the correct one to make. I had been so close to giving up several times but upon reflection now, I was very glad that I had been given the strength, the faith and the courage to continue to keep battling on. There had been a blood-stained crimson banner fluttering around me so many times, but I had not surrendered, nor had I given in.

I decided to continue with my other supplements, in addition to the immunotherapy treatment that I was now receiving. These included my daily Sillybum (Milk Thistle) capsules, to help keep my liver enzymes under control. I stopped the pancreatic enzymes, as I believed they were no longer necessary but that they had certainly served their purpose for me at the time.

I continued taking my daily IP6 capsules, as the recent research I discovered had shown that by adding these along with an antihistamine supplement, improved the efficiency of the immunotherapy treatment. I selected to add the antihistamine Zyrtec, to my daily list of additional supplements, which I took each morning.

Further research had also shown that the additional supplementation of in-season pomegranates and cranberries in conjunction with the Keytruda, had also shown even greater efficacy, in assisting the immunotherapy treatment to work even better.

This was featured in an article of the Science magazine in January 2018 and had been discovered by researchers from the University of Chicago in the United States. They had shown that specific strains of bacteria in the intestines improved the response rate of patients being treated for advanced metastatic melanoma cancer.

I continued with adding Resveratrol in various forms and I also kept avoiding sugars as much as possible. My daily intake of Fortisip compact protein was maintained, as well as a new supplementation of half a spoonful of pharmaceutical grade Creatine in a small glass of water each morning before breakfast.

I decided to order a book once again that I had originally been told about over twenty years ago, when I worked in a Department Store in Maroochydore on the Sunshine Coast in Queensland. One day in the store, a customer who was browsing stopped to have a chat with me. It turned out he was originally from a town called Killyleagh in Northern Ireland, which I knew well. I cannot remember how the conversation first started but I can probably relate it to my sales role in the kitchen and food department of the store.

He asked me if I had ever heard of a particular book called "Eat right for your type by Peter D'Amo." I said that "No, I hadn't and what was it about?" He then told me, it's a book written about people's individual blood groups and the diet that should be eaten by people who had a specific blood group. I found it very interesting, as I already knew my blood group was an "O Positive." I remembered purchasing the book at that time and reading it, however subsequently over the last twenty years, I had either managed to lose it or else I had lent it to others.

I searched for another copy of this old book, and I managed to find one online in the USA. I purchased the book, and I started reading it again, albeit twenty years later after the first purchase.

I found it strange, that in 2021 I had remembered this book and that I had started to eat this particular same diet once again and since then I can honestly say that my health has been in peak condition once more. The book stated that 'O' group people are carnivorous eaters. Maybe all those years earlier the stranger and the conversation about the book, was meant to happen. I restarted on my previous diet as up to this point I had cut out all meat and dairy products.

THE SUN SHINES AGAIN

My next treatment cycle was scheduled for the end of July 2021. This was to become my very last treatment in Brisbane before relocating from the Sunshine Coast to the Fraser Coast in Queensland. As this was going to become my last treatment cycle at this hospital, I decided to purchase a bottle of champagne as a gift for my good friend Trish, the nurse who had supported me during my entire period of attending this hospital. She had been there for me through both the good times, and through the very bad times, when I almost didn't make it. This treatment cycle went fine once again, and the infusion was completed inside sixty minutes, without any side effects. I then bade my farewells to the nursing staff, many of whom had been in their respective roles in the same department since my first shocking chemotherapy poisoning in 2011.

It was very sad to farewell Trish as she had supported me so much, as had all the other nurses in the cancer treatment rooms. I had always respected the nursing staff here as it was a very difficult and emotionally sad part of the hospital to have to work in each day, surrounded by so much sorrow.

I transferred hospitals at this stage to the Fraser Coast where I still continue to receive my treatment every six weeks, up to this point.

I continue to take my own supplements daily, as I firmly believe that my entire protocol, that I developed entirely myself, has been successful in helping me to rebuild again.

Since recommencing the immunotherapy, I have also started to develop an auto-immune condition called Vitiligo. This is a good sign that the treatment is continuing to work for me. The skin can develop a loss of colour from the body attacking the melanocytes. This means that anything the body can see relating to melanoma, it attacks.

I have also started personal training again each morning, which sadly, I had been unable to continue with during so much sickness.

A short time after commencing the Keytruda at the Fraser Coast, the new oncologist requested a recent PET scan. This was completed in October 2021. The results of the scan showed once more that there had been a very remarkable improvement in my health condition. There were no new tumours, and my body was almost totally clear of the melanoma cancer at this point. I still had two tumours left in my brain but they were rapidly shrinking from their original size of twenty-five millimetres down to ten millimetres. This was now seven years from I had received my three months left to live verdict, which had been delivered to me in October 2014.

It was certainly very clear to me now, that the treatment that I had been taken off in 2017 (which was another very blatant medical blunder) was indeed the correct treatment that I had originally selected for myself at that time.

It was now shown to have been very successful in helping my body's own immune system to reprogram itself to attack and destroy the pathogens, which are the cancer cell invaders.

I continued to have my quarterly brain scans carried out at Nambour on the Sunshine Coast, as the brain specialist who conducted my two previous Gamma Knife procedures preferred to have the images taken from the same scanning machine at that hospital for all his subsequent comparisons.

As of my writing now, which is December 2022, my last PET scan has shown, there are no tumours showing up on any of the scans.

My most recent MRI scan of my brain has also revealed that it's very likely that the two remaining tumours, which are around ten millimetres each, appear to be stable and are most likely now only to be old scar tissues left over from previously destroyed melanoma brain tumours.

At this stage I intend to continue with my existing immunotherapy treatment, and I will also continue with my own supplement regime. My brain specialist has also confirmed that he is now content to extend my regular quarterly brain scans to every four months instead of three months.

During my last telephone consultation with the same specialist, he said to me, "Rob, it just goes to show, that you were right all along the way, with the treatment that you selected for yourself."

I'm sure as you have already discovered from reading through my book, this has been a very long and difficult journey.

It's also been a very sad journey at times, to see so many of my other cancer friends travelling along the same pathway, who unfortunately have not been able to make it through to the end of their own journeys.

Thank you very much for purchasing my book. I think the moral of my story is very clear. Don't just simply accept everything that you have been told by so called specialists.

Always try to seek other opinions from those in a similar field if you're not sure, or if you are in any doubt or discomfort with what you have been told. Carry out your own research, ask for copies of your reports. If I had of known in 2010 what I know now, things would have been very different for me. Instead of having my life destroyed through medical mistakes.

I placed my total trust in the system, because like most people do, I didn't think I had any reason to disbelieve it, but the system failed me on so many occasions, that I almost lost my life. The fact that I was coerced into having unnecessary chemical poisoning in the first place, that destroyed my body's own immune system, when I didn't even have any signs of cancer showing in my body at that time, is very clear evidence of this.

The result being that I developed cancer from it. If you need to ask for a copy of your scans, your blood test results, or your Bone Marrow aspirates, then you should do it before giving your consent to anything that you feel uncomfortable with.

Even by doing this, the fact that it can also be so wrong at times, which happened to me losing my salivary gland after three needle aspirates confirmed it was suspicious of cancerous melanoma tumour and should be removed, when it turned out to be only a have been a fatty tissue cyst, unfortunately is further proof of this.

I hope that from reading my personal story that you found my cancer story interesting and informative and that it may just offer some hope, reassurance and help to others, who may have the misfortune of being on a similar pathway to the one I have been travelling.

<u>DON'T JUST GIVE UP</u>

I have been asked many times by others: -

"Rob, how do you manage to keep going with having a Terminal illness?"

I have always had two very simple 'mantras' in my life that I share with others, I usually reply with either one or both: -

"Places to be, people to see, that's me."

"In life we all have three choices that we can make,"

"We can either"

GIVE UP
GIVE IN or
GIVE IT ALL WE'VE GOT

The cells in your body react to everything that your mind says
Negativity brings down your immune system

Whenever you find yourself doubting if you can go on
Just remember how far you have come
Remember everything you have faced
All the battles you have won and all the fears you have overcome
Then raise your head up high and forge ahead knowing, that
You Got This!

When you face difficult times
Know that challenges are not sent to destroy you,
They are sent to promote, increase and strengthen you.

"Survive the dark and you will become the light"

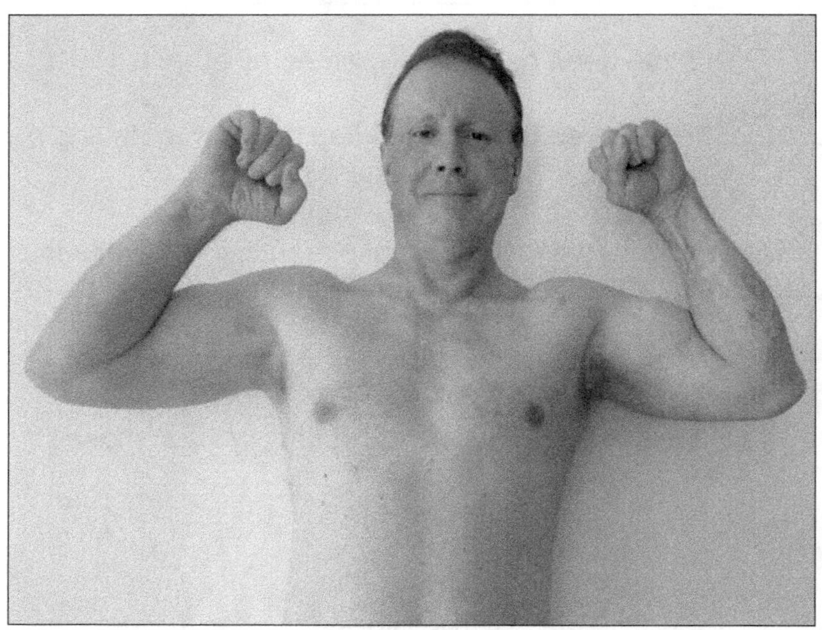

Robin December 2022

Thank you for reading my story.

I hope from reading it, that you might find the inspiration and courage to overcome the struggles and challenges that this disease presents to us each day and to never give up. There is always hope, even when at times it may feel to you that there is no hope left.

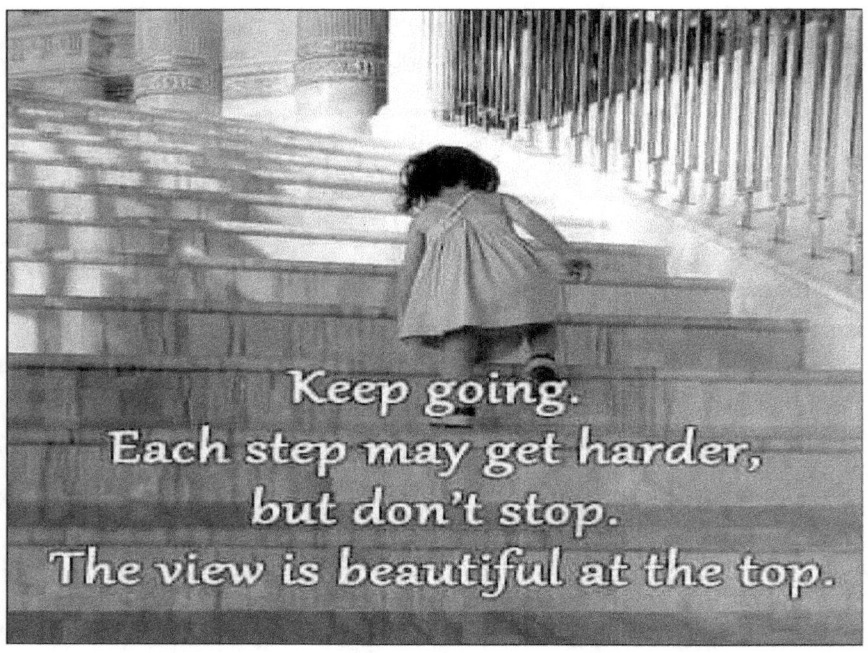